Contents

Introduction

Global Health is Volume 273 in the **ISSUES** series. The aim of the series is to offer current, diverse information about important issues in our world, from a UK perspective.

ABOUT GLOBAL HEALTH

The Millennium Development Goals aimed to halt and reverse the spread of HIV/AIDS, malaria and other major diseases by 2015. But with 2.3 million people newly infected with HIV and 207,000 cases of malaria in 2012, is this target likely to be achieved? This book explores the major diseases affecting our global health such as malaria, tuberculosis and, more recently, the Ebola virus. It also looks at the issue of sanitation and how this affects girls and women in particular, as well as how India managed to become free from polio in just five years.

OUR SOURCES

Titles in the **ISSUES** series are designed to function as educational resource books, providing a balanced overview of a specific subject.

The information in our books is comprised of facts, articles and opinions from many different sources, including:

⇨ Newspaper reports and opinion pieces

⇨ Website factsheets

⇨ Magazine and journal articles

⇨ Statistics and surveys

⇨ Government reports

⇨ Literature from special interest groups.

A NOTE ON CRITICAL EVALUATION

Because the information reprinted here is from a number of different sources, readers should bear in mind the origin of the text and whether the source is likely to have a particular bias when presenting information (or when conducting their research). It is hoped that, as you read about the many aspects of the issues explored in this book, you will critically evaluate the information presented.

It is important that you decide whether you are being presented with facts or opinions. Does the writer give a biased or unbiased report? If an opinion is being expressed, do you agree with the writer? Is there potential bias to the 'facts' or statistics behind an article?

ASSIGNMENTS

In the back of this book, you will find a selection of assignments designed to help you engage with the articles you have been reading and to explore your own opinions. Some tasks will take longer than others and there is a mixture of design, writing and research-based activities that you can complete alone or in a group.

FURTHER RESEARCH

At the end of each article we have listed its source and a website that you can visit if you would like to conduct your own research. Please remember to critically evaluate any sources that you consult and consider whether the information you are viewing is accurate and unbiased.

Useful weblinks

www.theconversation.com

www.deloitte.co.uk

www.downtoearth.org.

www.hscic.gov.uk Health & Social Care Information Centre

www.imperial.ac.uk

www.monash.edu

www.msf.org.uk Medecins Sans Frontieres

www.nhs.uk

www.polioeradication.org

www.savethechildren.org

www.toilettwinning.org

www.ucl.ac.uk University College London

www.unaids.org

www.unicef.org

www.warwick.ac.uk

www.wateraid.org

www.wellcome.ac.uk

www.who.int World Health Organization

www.world-heart-federation.org

www.yougov.co.uk

Global Health

Series Editor: Cara Acred

Volume 273

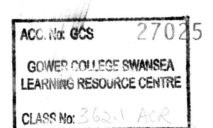
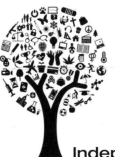

Independence Educational Publishers

First published by Independence Educational Publishers

The Studio, High Green

Great Shelford

Cambridge CB22 5EG

England

© Independence 2015

British Library Cataloguing in Publication Data

Global health. -- (Issues ; 273)

1. World health.

I. Series II. Acred, Cara editor.

362.1-dc23

ISBN-13: 9781861687012

Printed in Great Britain

Zenith Print Group

World Health Statistics 2014

Large gains in life expectancy.

People everywhere are living longer, according to the *World Health Statistics 2014* published today by WHO. Based on global averages, a girl who was born in 2012 can expect to live to around 73 years, and a boy to the age of 68. This is six years longer than the average global life expectancy for a child born in 1990.

WHO's annual statistics report shows that low-income countries have made the greatest progress, with an average increase in life expectancy by nine years from 1990 to 2012. The top six countries where life expectancy increased the most were Liberia which saw a 20-year increase (from 42 years in 1990 to 62 years in 2012) followed by Ethiopia (from 45 to 64 years), Maldives (58 to 77 years), Cambodia (54 to 72 years), Timor-Leste (50 to 66 years) and Rwanda (48 to 65 years).

'An important reason why global life expectancy has improved so much is that fewer children are dying before their fifth birthday,' says Dr Margaret Chan, WHO Director-General. 'But there is still a major rich-poor divide: people in high-income countries continue to have a much better chance of living longer than people in low-income countries.'

Gaps between rich and poor countries

A boy born in 2012 in a high-income country can expect to live to the age of around 76 – 16 years longer than

Life expectancy at birth among men and women in 2012 in the ten top-ranked countries					
Men			**Women**		
Rank	Country	Life expectancy	Rank	Country	Life expectancy
1	Iceland	81.2	1	Japan	87
2	Switzerland	80.7	2	Spain	85.1
3	Australia	80.5	3	Switzerland	85.1
4	Israel	80.2	4	Singapore	85.1
5	Singapore	80.2	5	Italy	85
6	New Zealand	80.2	6	France	84.9
7	Italy	80.2	7	Australia	84.6
8	Japan	80	8	Republic of Korea	84.6
9	Sweden	80	9	Luxembourg	84.1
10	Luxembourg	79.7	10	Portugal	84

a boy born in a low-income country (age 60). For girls, the difference is even wider; a gap of 19 years separates life expectancy in high-income (82 years) and low-income countries (63 years).

Wherever they live in the world, women live longer than men. The gap between male and female life expectancy is greater in high-income countries where women live around six years longer than men. In low-income countries, the difference is around three years.

Women in Japan have the longest life expectancy in the world at 87 years, followed by Spain, Switzerland and Singapore. Female life expectancy in all the top ten countries was 84 years or longer. Life expectancy among men is 80 years or more in nine countries, with the longest male life

expectancy in Iceland, Switzerland and Australia.

'In high-income countries, much of the gain in life expectancy is due to success in tackling noncommunicable diseases,' says Dr Ties Boerma, Director of the Department of Health Statistics and Information Systems at WHO. 'Fewer men and women are dying before they get to their 60th birthday from heart disease and stroke. Richer countries have become better at monitoring and managing high blood pressure for example.'

Declining tobacco use is also a key factor in helping people live longer in several countries.

At the other end of the scale, life expectancy for both men and women is still less than 55 years in nine sub-Saharan African countries – Angola,

Central African Republic, Chad, Côte d'Ivoire, Democratic Republic of the Congo, Lesotho, Mozambique, Nigeria and Sierra Leone.

Some other key facts from World Health Statistics 2014

⇨ The top three causes of years of life lost due to premature death are coronary heart disease, lower respiratory infections (such as pneumonia) and stroke.

⇨ Worldwide, a major shift is occurring in the causes and ages of death. In 22 countries (all in Africa), 70% or more of years of life lost (due to premature deaths) are still caused by infectious diseases and related conditions. Meanwhile, in 47 countries (mostly high-income), noncommunicable diseases and injuries cause more than 90% of years of life lost. More than 100 countries are transitioning rapidly towards a greater proportion of deaths from noncommunicable diseases and injuries.

⇨ Around 44 million (6.7%) of the world's children aged less than five years were overweight or obese in 2012. Ten million of these children were in the WHO African Region where levels of child obesity have increased rapidly.

⇨ Most deaths among under-fives occur among children born prematurely (17.3%); pneumonia is responsible for the second highest number of deaths (15.2%).

⇨ Between 1995 and 2012, 56 million people were successfully treated for tuberculosis and 22 million lives were saved. In 2012, an estimated 450,000 people worldwide developed multi-drug resistant tuberculosis.

⇨ Only one-third of all deaths worldwide are recorded in civil registries along with cause-of-death information.

15 May 2014

⇨ The above information is reprinted with kind permission from the World Health Organization. Please visit www.who.int for further information.

World Health Statistics 2014

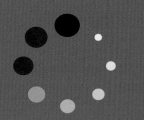

Between 2000 and 2012, measles deaths worldwide have been cut by almost 80% – from 562,000 to 122,000 deaths.

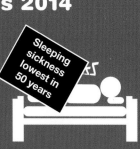

Human African trypanosomiasis (commonly known as sleeping sickness) is at its lowest level in 50 years, with fewer than 10,000 cases of infection reported in 2009.

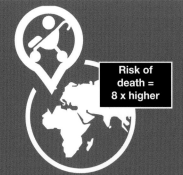

The risk of a child dying before their fifth birthday is eight times higher in the WHO African Region than a child in the WHO European Region.

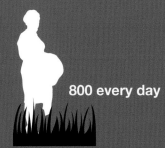

800 every day

Nearly 800 women die every day due to complications in pregnancy and childbirth.

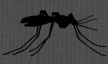

More than 2.5 million people worldwide are estimated to be at risk of dengue infection.

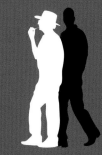

In the WHO Western Pacific Region, almost one in two adult men smoke tobacco.

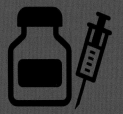

In 2012, more than 140,000 people in high-income countries had pertussis (whooping cough), a serious disease in infants that is preventable by vaccination.

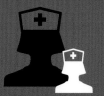

High-income countries have an average of almost 90 nurses and midwives for every 10,000 people while some low-income countries have fewer than two per 10,000 people.

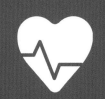

The top three causes of premature death are coronary heart disease, lower respiratory infections and stroke.

2014 Global healthcare sector outlook

Among drivers for growth in the global health care sector are an ageing population, rising incidence of chronic diseases, increasing access to care; technological advancements and product innovation; and emerging market growth. Yet healthcare organisations also must address major issues in 2014 like navigating the impact of healthcare reforms in many countries; rising costs; quality issues; lack of infrastructure in many parts of the world; workforce issues; and safety and privacy concerns. The challenges and opportunities emanating from each of these areas can be both global and market-specific.

'The shared, long-term trends of an ageing population and an increase in people inflicted with chronic diseases are expected to drive demand for healthcare services'

Issue #1: ageing population and rise of chronic disease

The shared, long-term trends of an ageing population and an increase in people inflicted with chronic diseases are expected to drive demand for healthcare services in both developed and emerging economies in 2014 and beyond. The ageing population, which is expected to more than triple again over the next half-century, and increasing life expectancies are expected to place a huge burden on the healthcare system in many markets. Another shared demographic trend creating increased healthcare demand is the spread of chronic diseases – heart disease, stroke, cancer, chronic respiratory diseases, diabetes and mental illness, among others – which are, by far, the leading cause of mortality in the world, representing 63 per cent of all deaths, and can be attributable to the ageing population, more sedentary lifestyles, diet changes, and rising obesity levels, as well as improved diagnostics.

Issue #2: cost and quality

Whether a country is spending nearly 18 per cent GDP on health care (like the U.S.) or recession-riddled Europe, which is spending around ten per cent, public and private funding systems are economically stressed – across the globe, rising costs are unaffordable and unsustainable. Healthcare cost increases can be attributed to numerous factors, such as industry consolidation, prolonged hospital stays, expensive biologics and diagnostics which are outpacing traditional therapies, inefficient processes, and overuse of medicines. Unfortunately, higher costs do not necessarily correlate to better results or higher-quality care, even in developed countries. Sometimes, the biggest danger to patients is not their disease but the hospitals that treat them.

Issue #3: access to care

Improving healthcare access is a major goal of governments around the world, and a centrepiece of many reform efforts in many countries. While facilitating increased healthcare access is an important and worthy endeavour, more people in the system means more demand for services that numerous healthcare systems are unable to accommodate due to workforce shortages, patient locations, and infrastructure limitations, in addition to the cost issues identified earlier. Many countries across the globe are facing a challenge to meet their required number of healthcare workers, a shortage that directly affects the quality of care. Uneven distribution of caregivers is also a problem. Patient location can be another deterrent to care. A third constraint on patient access is lack of healthcare infrastructure in certain countries and outdated facilities in both developed and emerging markets.

'Across the world, healthcare systems are recognising the need for innovation'

Issue #4: technology

Across the world, healthcare systems are recognising the need for innovation; advances in health technologies and data management can help facilitate new diagnostic and treatment options; however, these same advances are likely to increase overall costs, prompting widespread efforts by public and private healthcare providers and insurers to contain expenditure by restructuring care delivery models and promoting more efficient use of resources. Healthcare technology changes will be rapid and, in some parts of the world, disruptive to established health care models. Yet, acquiring and leveraging technology innovations require financial investments that many healthcare providers – even in developed economies – may struggle to afford in an era of cost-cutting and reform. The technology-enabled, transforming healthcare system is producing an immense volume of information and, more specifically, how to interpret and use that data will be important. Much rides upon its availability, integrity and confidentiality. Potential patient safety, economic and reputational damage may also arise if organisations lack appropriate security and privacy controls.

⇨ The above information is reprinted with kind permission from Deloitte. Please visit www.deloitte.co.uk for further information.

AIDS by the numbers

Latest estimates from the Joint United Nations Programme on HIV/AIDS (UNAIDS) show that the world continues to close in on the goal of ending the AIDS epidemic by stopping HIV transmission and halting AIDS-related deaths. Remarkable progress has been made over the last decade – yet significant challenges remain.

New HIV infections

Globally, the number of new HIV infections continues to fall. There were 2.3 million new HIV infections [1.9 million–2.7 million] in 2012. This is the lowest number of annual new infections since the mid-to-late 1990s, when approximately 3.5 million [3.3 million–4.1 million] people were acquiring HIV every year.

The number of HIV infections declined by more than 50% in 26 countries between 2001 and 2002 and between 25% and 49% in an additional 17 countries.

The drop in new HIV infections is most pronounced among children. From 2001 to 2012 the number of children newly infected with HIV dropped by 52% – from 550,000 [500,000–620,000] in 2001 to 260,000 [230,000–320,000] in 2012.

Access to treatment

The cost of first line antiretroviral therapy in some low-and-middle-income countries has been reduced to around US$140 per person per year. In the mid-1990s, the cost was around US$10,000 per person per year.

Increased political commitment and smarter investments, together with more strategic programming and massive reductions in the cost of treatment have led to a record 9.7 million people in low- and middle-income countries having access to antiretroviral therapy at the end of 2012. The rate of scale up has increased exponentially in recent years. In 2012 alone an additional 1.6 million people newly gained access to treatment.

A major advance in expanding access to treatment has been the scientific discovery that initiating treatment earlier will save more lives. In 2013, the World Health Organization (WHO) amended its guidelines based on this new evidence to recommend that treatment is started much earlier, and immediately in some cases. This means that 28.6 million [26.5–30.9 million] people were eligible for treatment in 2013.

Science has also shown that if pregnant women living with HIV have access to antiretroviral medicines the risk of transmitting the virus to their child can be reduced to below 5%. As a result, access has dramatically increased. By 2012, some 62% of pregnant women living with HIV had access to antiretroviral medicines and in many countries coverage levels exceeded 80%.

AIDS-related deaths

The massive scale up of antiretroviral therapy is saving more lives. The number of people dying from AIDS-related causes each year has declined from a high of 2.3 million [2.1–2.6 million] in 2005 to 1.6 million [1.4–1.9 million] in 2012.

Since 2004, TB-related deaths among people living with HIV have declined by 36% world-wide.

HIV and aging

Out of the global total of 35.3 million [32.2 million–38.8 million] people living with HIV, an estimated 3.6 million [3.2 million–3.9 million] are people aged 50 years or older.

The majority – 2.9 million [2.6 million–3.1 million] – are in low- and middle-income countries where the percentage of adults living with HIV who are 50 years or older is now above 10%. In high-income countries around one third of adults living with HIV are 50 years or older.

Sexual behaviours are becoming less safe in some countries

There are signs of an increase in risky sexual behaviours in several countries. Recent evidence indicates a significant increase in the number of sexual partners in some countries (Burkina Faso, Congo, Cote d'Ivoire, Ethiopia, Gabon, Guyana, Rwanda, South Africa, Uganda, the United Republic of Tanzania and Zimbabwe), as well as a decline in condom use (in Cote d'Ivoire, Niger, Senegal and Uganda).

Persistent challenges to effective HIV prevention efforts for adolescents and young people include inadequate access to high-quality, youth-friendly HIV and sexual and reproductive education and health services, and sexual violence against young women and girls.

Access to HIV treatment

Under the 2013 WHO guidelines, the HIV treatment coverage in low- and middle-income countries represented only 34% (32–37%) of the 28.6 million people eligible in 2013.

To start treatment people need to know their HIV status. Globally it is estimated that only around half of all people living with HIV know their HIV status. Once linked to care there are mixed feelings regarding retention. According to data from 18 countries, retention in HIV care declines over time, with 12- and 60-month retention rates of 86% and 72%, respectively.

Children living with HIV continue to experience persistent treatment gaps. In 2012, 647,000 children under 15 years of age were receiving antiretroviral treatment. HIV treatment coverage for children remained half of coverage for adults in 2012.

2013

⇨ The above information is reprinted with kind permission from UNAIDS. Please visit www.unaids.org for further information.

TB rises in UK and London

London is 'the TB capital of Europe', *The Daily Telegraph* has reported. The newspaper says that Britain is now the only nation in Western Europe with rising levels of tuberculosis, with more than 9,000 cases diagnosed annually. In London, where 40% of UK cases are reportedly diagnosed, the number of cases has risen by almost 50% since 1999, up from 2,309 in 1999 to 3,450 in 2009.

The Guardian has also discussed the rising prevalence of the disease, which was detailed in a report on the modern TB situation in London, as well as the UK as a whole. The report's author, Professor Alimuddin Zumla of University College London, attributes the rise to people living under 'Victorian' conditions, with poor housing, inadequate ventilation and overcrowding in certain deprived areas of London.

Professor Zumla has also observed that the increase in TB cases has been predominantly among people born outside the UK, but who appear to have been infected here, rather than in their country of origin. He has called for the implementation of a London-wide strategy to help control the disease.

What is tuberculosis?

Tuberculosis is a disease caused by the bacterium *Mycobacterium tuberculosis*.

Infection predominantly affects the lungs, though it can spread via the blood to affect other organs. Like other respiratory infections, TB is spread by airborne droplets passed on through sneezing and coughing. It is mostly spread through prolonged contact with an infected person. TB differs from other airborne infections such as colds and flu in that it is not typically passed on by short-term contact, such as when using public transport.

When initially infected, a person may have no symptoms and can remain without symptoms for a long time. However, if the person's immune system is weak, the infection can progress to active disease and the person is likely to develop:

⇨ a persistent productive cough that brings up sputum or phlegm, which may contain blood

⇨ fever and sweating

⇨ general symptoms of illness, such as fatigue

⇨ weight loss.

As such, the symptoms of TB need to be distinguished from those of chronic bronchitis, pneumonia or cancer, which are similar. The disease is usually diagnosed using X-rays and laboratory examination of sputum samples, and is treated with a combination of antibiotics over a prolonged period of at least six months.

Tuberculosis is known to occur more often in areas of deprivation, where poor living conditions, poor nutrition and poorer health are more common. Those with a depleted immune system and poorer general health are at increased risk; for example, people with HIV, alcoholics and those who are malnourished.

What is the basis for the current reports?

The news stories follow a narrative review authored by Professor Alimuddin Zumla, a consultant in infectious disease at University College London Hospital and the director of the Centre for Infectious Diseases and International Health at University College London Medical School. The review was published in *The Lancet* medical journal.

Professor Zumla discusses the history and resurgence of what was known in the Victorian times as consumption, or 'the white plague', due to the pale complexion of sufferers. In the 1800s up to 25% of deaths in Europe were attributed to TB. In the 1900s, however, improved housing, nutrition and economic status brought a decline in prevalence, which was then reduced greatly by the advent of anti-tuberculosis drugs in the 1960s.

By the 1980s, TB was considered to be almost eradicated in the UK. However, this is said to have changed again with the increase in travel and migration. The review suggests that the poorer socio-economic status and living conditions experienced by certain population groups have led to a gradual re-emergence of TB as a public health problem in Europe.

The review gives an overview of the modern toll of TB, saying that:

⇨ Currently 1.7 million people die of tuberculosis globally each year.

⇨ Incidence in the UK has gradually increased over the past 15 years, with more than 9,000 cases reported in 2009, a rate of 14.6 per 100,000 population. This is said to contrast with a general decline seen in other western European countries, with the UK being the only European country where TB rates continue to rise.

⇨ In London, the number of cases has risen by almost 50% since 1999, up from 2,309 in 1999 to 3,450 in 2009. London now accounts for almost 40% of all TB cases in the UK.

⇨ The increase in the number of tuberculosis cases in the UK has largely been in non-UK born groups. In 2009, these included black African (28%), Indian (27%) and white people (10%). However, 85% of individuals born overseas had lived in the UK for at least two years prior to being diagnosed, i.e. they were not recent immigrants. This suggests transmission may have occurred after they had arrived in the UK.

⇨ Poor living conditions are known to be associated with TB and, in particular, the author considers prisons to be 'ideal breeding grounds'. He quotes a four-year study (2004–07) of 205 prisoners with newly-diagnosed TB that demonstrated that, compared with all other cases in the UK during that period (29,340 in total), prisoners were more likely to be UK born (47% versus 25%) and to be white (33% versus 22%). Only 48% of prisoners diagnosed with active disease completed treatment, and 20% were lost to follow-up.

As the current figures reflect only reported cases, the true disease prevalence may be even higher. The narrative highlights the need for healthcare professionals in the UK, and particularly London, to have heightened awareness of TB as a possible cause of disease in their patients in order to improve diagnosis. The author also raises the problem of antibiotic resistance that has been observed in certain cases over the past ten years, particularly those occurring among people in prison. This highlights the need for people to complete full courses of antibiotic treatment.

What does the author conclude?

The author says that the current situation in London has similarities with previous outbreaks of drug-resistant TB in the US in the 1990s, where a large amount of financial investment and government support was required to regain control of the disease through the clear establishment of clinical policy and protocol.

The author also says that there is now a need to implement the recommendations of a recent London tuberculosis service review, which has suggested steps such as standardising the various testing and treatment methods used in different areas.

What else do I need to know about TB?

The BCG (Bacillus Calmette-Guerin) vaccination exposes the person to a weakened *Mycobacterium* strain, causing them to develop immunity against TB. In the UK the vaccine is no longer given routinely, but is given to those expected to be at higher risk of disease, which includes certain professionals (for example, healthcare workers, and people working in homeless shelters and refuge hostels), immigrants coming to the UK from high-incidence areas and infants born into high-incidence areas such as inner London or whose parents come from high-incidence areas.

Anyone with a cough, productive or not, that has persisted for more than a few weeks should consult their doctor, as should any person with feverish symptoms, unexplained weight loss, general fatigue and loss of appetite. These could be signs not only of TB, but of other serious illness.

As stated, TB is a curable disease, as long as a prolonged course of antibiotics is followed. However, as with any antibiotic treatment, failing to complete a full course can lead to the development of antibiotic resistant strains of bacteria.

Tuberculosis is a 'notifiable disease' and, by law, government authorities must be informed of any cases identified. This information is gathered by the UK Health Protection Agency, which says that around 9,000 cases of TB are reported each year in the UK, with most cases occurring in major cities, particularly London. The HPA says it is committed to supporting the NHS and the Department of Health in controlling TB in the UK.

17 December 2013

⇨ The above information is reprinted with kind permission from NHS Choices. Please visit www.nhs.uk for further information.

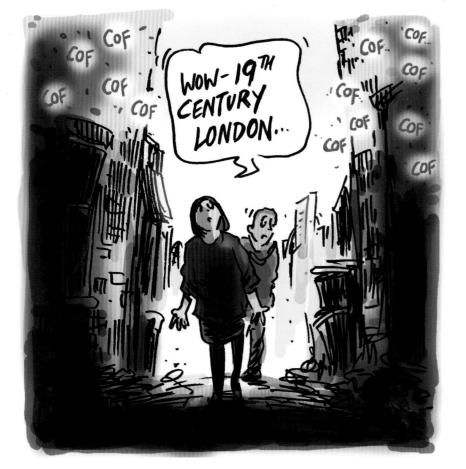

Tuberculosis is an old disease with a new face – and it needs to be stopped

When rich countries eradicated TB, new treatments dried up. Now the disease has evolved to become drug-resistant – and it's the world's poorest people who are bearing the brunt.

My role as a doctor is to make it possible for Andile to play football again. He used to train three times a week in Khayelitsha, one of the largest townships in South Africa – miles and miles of little brick houses interspaced with tin shacks on the edge of Cape Town. He says he was the type of player who didn't waste himself running aimlessly after the ball; rather, he analysed the game to make decisive passes that would lead his team to victory. But today, what Andile wishes above all is to be able to run, even aimlessly.

As it is, he can't even walk ten metres without having to bend over to catch his breath. His lungs are so weak he is unable even to laugh. Tuberculosis has devoured them.

TB is a very old disease. It used to be called phthisis, or consumption. It kills 1.5 million people every year and ranks right behind HIV as the world's biggest infectious killer. Since it all but disappeared in most of the richest parts of the world half a century ago, though, developments in new TB treatments ground to a halt. This has allowed plenty of time for one of humankind's most vicious enemies to develop ways to beat the defences that were engineered to fight it.

Nearly half a million people across the globe are infected by strains of tuberculosis against which existing drugs are powerless. In South Africa, where I work, 15,000 people were diagnosed as having drug-resistant TB (DR-TB) in 2012. Up to 80% of them caught it by unknowingly breathing it.

When they become ill, they come to see me. At those moments, I wish I had chosen to become a schoolteacher or a city planner or engineer – surely, in such professions I would be able to make a bigger difference to people's lives.

What am I to tell my patients? That, yes, we just celebrated the cure of 30-year-old Siyabulela, but that he is one of only four patients I have treated to beat extensively drug-resistant tuberculosis (XDR-TB), which jumps to its next victim every time someone infected sneezes? That the three other people who started the same treatment at the same time are long dead?

I can't bear having to look someone in the eye and tell them that I cannot give them better odds of survival than a roll of a dice. Roll a six, you'll live; if not, you'll be dead within two years. In South Africa, only 13% of XDR-TB patients are cured by the existing treatment regimen.

I also have to tell them that, for that slim shot at survival, they will have to endure a harrowing two years of treatment. For at least the first six months, they will receive daily injections that hurt so much they will be unable to sit down, and the injected drugs could make them permanently deaf. So limited is the medical arsenal at my disposal, another drug I may be forced to prescribe might trigger mental instability, causing psychotic episodes so acute that they could be a danger to themselves. But, I have to explain to my patients, they will only know after two years whether it was all worth it; only then will it become clear whether their roll of the dice produced the required six.

I'm sick and tired of using plasters to patch up gaping wounds. I need something I can really work with, something that can save lives. We need a new treatment regimen against TB that actually works. Treatment that has not been dredged up from the dark ages of modern medicine and reused because, well, it's better than nothing.

There is some hope on the horizon. For the first time in 50 years, new drugs are being developed to treat TB. They represent great strides forward, but they can't be used in isolation. TB is so powerful that you need a full cocktail of drugs to beat it. The only way to beat this disease is for governments, donors, pharmaceutical firms and research organisations to find new combinations of drugs that are simple, accessible and more tolerable than current treatment and can be implemented rapidly in countries where DR-TB is rife.

But by the time that dream is realised, 80% of the patients I see every day, who see my white doctor's coat as a life jacket, will be dead and gone, forgotten by all but their devastated families in the poorest corners of the country.

27 March 2014

⇨ The above information is reprinted with kind permission from *The Guardian*. Please visit www.theguardian.com for further information.

Over 50 million children infected with tuberculosis

A new study quantifying the global burden of tuberculosis among children suggests there are tens of millions of children with undiagnosed TB.

By Francesca Davenport

Researchers at the University of Sheffield, Imperial College London, and TB Alliance found evidence that there is a large gap between the number of recorded TB cases and the true incidence. The study, published today in *Lancet Global Health*, shows that TB in children is a major public health problem worldwide.

'In [...] 22 countries more than 650,000 children developed the disease in 2010, while 7.6 million became infected with the TB bacterium'

The investigators estimated the number of children with TB in the 22 countries with the highest burden of TB in the world using a mechanistic mathematical model. In contrast with standard estimates that are reliant on paediatric case reporting, which varies widely between countries, the researchers took a complementary approach, using mathematical modelling to estimate rates of infection and disease in children based on country-specific data on household and population structure, and the prevalence of TB in adults. The model incorporated both social and epidemiological variables including the effects of age, BCG vaccination efficacy, and the effect of HIV infection.

The study suggests that in these 22 countries more than 650,000 children developed the disease in 2010, while 7.6 million became infected with the TB bacterium. Overall more than 53 million children were estimated to harbour a latent infection.

Diagnosing TB in children can be challenging and the disease can often be overlooked or mistaken for something else. This can lead to under-reporting, distorting the true scope of the problem and the real demand for paediatric TB treatment.

The first estimates of paediatric TB by the World Health Organization (WHO) were published in 2012, and last year the WHO estimated 530,000 paediatric cases worldwide. However, given the acknowledged difficulties in detecting TB in children, there is need for additional research and focus on the burden of disease in children.

Health economics researcher Peter Dodd, from the University of Sheffield's School of Health and Related Research (ScHARR), said: 'Quantifying the burden of TB in children is important because, without good numbers, there can be no targets for improvement, no monitoring of trends and there is a lack of evidence to encourage industry to invest in developing medicines or diagnostics that are more appropriate for children than those available today.'

He added: 'Historically, TB in children has not received the attention that it might have done. The WHO is now encouraging countries to report the number of TB cases they find in children, but we still have only a poor idea what proportion of cases are recorded in youngsters.'

The 22 countries with high TB investigated in the study are reported to harbour 80 per cent of the global burden. In addition to providing global estimates, the study also suggests that over a quarter of all paediatric TB cases were in India and 15 million children under the age of 15 were living with somebody who had TB. The 53 million children with latent TB represent a huge reservoir for future disease.

'Overall more than 53 million children were estimated to harbour a latent infection'

Co-author of the study, Dr James Seddon from the Department of Medicine, Imperial College London, said: 'Although these 53 million infected children may not be currently experiencing any problems, they are at a very high risk of developing the disease in the future. It is also interesting to note that only a third of children with TB disease are currently identified, treated and reported. This compares to two thirds in adults.'

The study is part of a larger effort, led by TB Alliance and supported by UNITAID and USAID, to improve TB treatment for children and deliver optimised child-friendly first-line TB drugs.

Reference: Dodd et al. 'Burden of childhood tuberculosis in 22 high-burden countries: a mathematical modelling study' 2014 *Lancet Global Health* http://www.thelancet.com/journals/langlo/article/PIIS2214-109X(14)70245-1/abstract

9 July 2014

⇨ The above information is reprinted with kind permission from Imperial College London. Please visit www.imperial.ac.uk for further information.

Polio and prevention

Polio is a crippling and potentially fatal infectious disease. There is no cure, but there are safe and effective vaccines. The strategy to eradicate polio is therefore based on preventing infection by immunising every child until transmission stops and the world is polio-free.

The disease

Polio (poliomyelitis) is a highly infectious disease caused by a virus. It invades the nervous system and can cause irreversible paralysis in a matter of hours.

Who is at risk?

Polio can strike at any age, but it mainly affects children under five years old.

Transmission

Polio is spread through person-to-person contact. When a child is infected with wild poliovirus, the virus enters the body through the mouth and multiplies in the intestine. It is then shed into the environment through the faeces where it can spread rapidly through a community, especially in situations of poor hygiene and sanitation. If a sufficient number of children are fully immunised against polio, the virus is unable to find susceptible children to infect, and dies out.

Young children who are not yet toilet-trained are a ready source of transmission, regardless of their environment. Polio can be spread when food or drink is contaminated by faeces. There is also evidence that flies can passively transfer poliovirus from faeces to food.

Most people infected with the poliovirus have no signs of illness and are never aware they have been infected. These symptomless people carry the virus in their intestines and can 'silently' spread the infection to thousands of others before the first case of polio paralysis emerges.

For this reason, WHO considers a single confirmed case of polio paralysis to be evidence of an epidemic – particularly in countries where very few cases occur.

Symptoms

Most infected people (90%) have no symptoms or very mild symptoms and usually go unrecognised. In others, initial symptoms include fever, fatigue, headache, vomiting, stiffness in the neck and pain in the limbs.

Acute flaccid paralysis (AFP)

One in 200 infections leads to irreversible paralysis, usually in the legs. This is caused by the virus entering the bloodstream and invading the central nervous system. As it multiplies, the virus destroys the nerve cells that activate muscles. The affected muscles are no longer functional and the limb becomes floppy and lifeless – a condition known as acute flaccid paralysis (AFP).

All cases of acute flaccid paralysis (AFP) among children under 15 years of age are reported and tested for poliovirus within 48 hours of onset.

Bulbar polio

More extensive paralysis, involving the trunk and muscles of the thorax and abdomen, can result in quadriplegia. In the most severe cases (bulbar polio), poliovirus attacks the nerve cells of the brain stem, reducing breathing capacity and causing difficulty in swallowing and speaking. Among those paralysed, 5% to 10% die when their breathing muscles become immobilised.

Post-polio syndrome

Around 40% of people who survive paralytic polio may develop additional symptoms 15–40 years after the original illness. These symptoms – called post-polio syndrome – include new progressive muscle weakness, severe fatigue and pain in the muscles and joints.

Risk factors for paralysis

No one knows why only a small percentage of infections lead to paralysis. Several key risk factors have been identified as increasing the likelihood of paralysis in a person infected with polio. These include:

⇨ immune deficiency

⇨ pregnancy

⇨ removal of the tonsils (tonsillectomy)

⇨ intramuscular injections, e.g. medications

⇨ strenuous exercise

⇨ injury.

Treatment and prevention

There is no cure for polio, only treatment to alleviate the symptoms. Heat and physical therapy is used to stimulate the muscles and antispasmodic drugs are given to relax the muscles. While this can improve mobility, it cannot reverse permanent polio paralysis.

Polio can be prevented through immunisation. Polio vaccine, given multiple times, almost always protects a child for life.

⇨ The above information is reprinted with kind permission from the World Health Organization. Please visit www.polioeradication.org for further information.

© The Global Polio Eradication Initiative 2014

What is Ebola virus?

Ebola virus disease is a serious, usually fatal, disease for which there are no licensed treatments or vaccines. But for people living in countries outside Africa, it remains a very low threat.

Ebola was first identified in Africa in the mid-1970s. An outbreak that began in March 2014 was the most serious so far. By 13 August 2014 it had killed more than 1,000 people across Guinea, Liberia, Sierra Leone and Nigeria.

In August 2014, a British nurse who was treating patients in Sierra Leone contracted the Ebola virus and was flown back to the UK for treatment in a London hospital. But experts studying the virus believe it is very unlikely the disease will spread within the UK.

How do Ebola outbreaks start?

It's thought the Ebola virus has been living harmlessly in fruit bats for many years, building up in this population and spreading to other forest animals including chimpanzees and gorillas.

It's likely the virus makes its way into people after they butcher or handle dead animals contaminated with the virus.

How does it spread among people?

People can become infected with the Ebola virus if they come into contact with the blood, body fluids or organs of an infected person.

Most people are infected by giving care to other infected people, either by directly touching the victim's body or by cleaning up body fluids (stools, urine or vomit) that carry infectious blood.

Traditional African burial rituals have also played a part in its spread. The Ebola virus can survive for several days outside the body, including on the skin of an infected person, and it's common practice for mourners to touch the body of the deceased. They only then need to touch their mouth to become infected.

Other ways people can catch Ebola are:

⇨ touching the soiled clothing of an infected person, then touching their mouth

⇨ having sex with an infected person without using a condom (the virus is present in semen for up to seven weeks after the infected person has recovered)

⇨ handling unsterilised needles or medical equipment that were used in the care of the infected person.

The person is infectious as long as their blood, urine, stools or secretions contain the virus.

Ebola virus disease is generally not spread through routine social contact (such as shaking hands) with patients who do not have symptoms.

The virus is not, for example, as infectious as diseases like the flu, as airborne transmission is much less likely. You'd need to have close contact with the source of infection to be at risk.

Who is at risk?

Anyone who cares for an infected person or handles their blood or fluid samples is at risk of becoming infected. Hospital workers, laboratory workers and family members are at greatest risk.

Strict infection control procedures and wearing protective clothing minimises this risk – see 'What's the advice for healthcare and aid workers?' below. Simply washing hands with soap and water can destroy the virus.

What are the symptoms?

An infected person will typically develop a fever, headache, joint and muscle pain, sore throat, and intense muscle weakness. These symptoms start suddenly, between two and 21 days after becoming infected, but usually after five to seven days.

Diarrhoea, vomiting, a rash, stomach pain and impaired kidney and liver function follow.

The patient then bleeds internally, and may also bleed from the ears, eyes, nose or mouth.

Ebola virus disease is fatal in 50-90% of cases. The sooner a person is given care, the better the chances that they will survive.

How is it treated?

There's currently no licensed treatment or vaccine for Ebola virus disease, although potential new vaccines and drug therapies are being developed and tested.

Patients need to be placed in isolation in intensive care. Dehydration is common, so fluids may be given directly into a vein (intravenously). Blood oxygen levels and blood pressure need to be maintained at the right level and body organs supported while the patient's body fights the disease and any other infections are treated.

ZMapp is an experimental treatment that can be tried, although it has not yet been tested in humans for safety or effectiveness. The product is a combination of three different antibodies that bind to the protein of the Ebola virus.

What's the advice for healthcare and aid workers?

Any area affected by an outbreak should be immediately quarantined and patients treated in isolation.

Healthcare workers need to avoid contact with the bodily fluids of their infected patients by taking the following precautions:

⇨ wear face masks, goggles, gowns and gloves

⇨ take extra care when handling blood, secretions and catheters and when connecting patients to a drip

⇨ disinfect non-disposable medical equipment before re-use

⇨ sterilise and dispose of used needles and disposable equipment carefully

⇨ properly dispose of any secretions or body waste from the patient

⇨ carefully and frequently wash hands with soap and water

(alcohol hand rub if soap isn't available)

⇨ wash disposable gloves with soap and water after use, dispose of them carefully, then wash hands.

What's the advice for travellers in at-risk areas?

Following these simple precautions will minimise your risk of catching Ebola virus disease:

⇨ don't handle dead animals or their raw meat

⇨ don't eat 'bushmeat'

⇨ avoid contact with patients who have symptoms

⇨ avoid having sex with people in risk areas; use a condom if you do

⇨ make sure fruit and veg is washed and peeled before you eat it

⇨ wash hands frequently using soap and water (alcohol hand rubs when soap is not available), as this destroys the virus.

If you think you or a family member has symptoms of Ebola infection:

⇨ visit a healthcare provider immediately and inform them that you may have had contact with the Ebola virus (the nearest Embassy or Consular Office can help you find a provider in the area)

⇨ limit contact with others and avoid all other travel.

It's more likely that the cause is another disease such as malaria, but you may need to be tested for Ebola as a precaution.

What if I think I might have Ebola in the UK?

If you feel unwell with symptoms such as fever, chills, muscle aches, headache, nausea, vomiting, diarrhoea, sore throat or rash within 21 days of coming back from Guinea, Liberia or Sierra Leone, you should stay at home and immediately telephone 111 or 999 and explain that you have recently visited West Africa.

These services will provide advice and arrange for you to be seen in a hospital if necessary so the cause of your illness can be determined.

There are other illnesses that are much more common than Ebola (such as flu, typhoid fever and malaria) that have similar symptoms in the early stages, so proper medical assessment is really important to ensure you get the right diagnosis and treatment.

It is also really important that medical services are expecting your arrival and calling 111 or 999 will ensure this happens.

How is it diagnosed?

It's difficult to know if a patient is infected with Ebola virus in the early stages as symptoms such as fever, headache and muscle pain are similar to those of many other diseases.

But specialist infection clinicians will make expert judgements on what the most likely diagnosis is based on the patient's history.

If Ebola is considered a possibility on this basis, then a person would be tested for the disease.

Samples of blood or body fluid can be sent to a laboratory to be tested for the presence of Ebola virus, and a diagnosis can be made rapidly.

A suspect case would be isolated in a side room so as to minimise contacts with other people while they are being tested. It is only if this test is positive that the case is considered to be 'confirmed'.

If the test is positive then they will be transferred to a hospital-based high-level isolation unit.

If the result is negative, doctors will test for other diseases such as malaria, typhoid fever and cholera.

Why is the risk low for people in the UK?

The likelihood of catching Ebola virus disease is considered very low unless you've travelled to a known infected area and had direct contact with a person with Ebola-like symptoms, or had contact with an infected animal or contaminated objects.

There has been just one imported case of Ebola in the UK. While it is possible that more people infected with Ebola could arrive in the UK on a plane, the virus is not as easily transmitted as a respiratory virus such as influenza.

In past outbreaks, infection control measures have been very effective in containing Ebola within the immediate area. The UK has a robust public health system with the trained staff and facilities necessary to contain cases of Ebola.

Advice has been issued to the Border Force to identify possible cases of Ebola and there are procedures in place to provide care to the patient and to minimise public health risk to others.

Also, Ebola victims do not become infectious until shortly before they develop symptoms. The disease then progresses very rapidly. This means infectious people do not walk around spreading the disease for a long period.

It typically takes five to seven days for symptoms to develop after infection, so there is time to identify people who may have been exposed, put them under surveillance and if they show symptoms, quarantine them.

Flight crew are trained to respond swiftly to any passengers who develop symptoms during a flight from Africa. They will take measures to reduce transmission on board the plane. But this event is very unlikely, and so far there have been no documented cases of people catching the disease simply by being in the same plane as an Ebola victim.

I may have been on a flight with someone with Ebola. Am I at risk?

You cannot catch Ebola through social contact or by travelling on a plane with someone who is infected, without direct contact with the blood or body fluids of an infected person.

Cabin crew identifying a sick passenger with suspicion of infectious disease on board, as well as ground staff receiving the passenger at the destination, would follow the International Air

Transport Association guidelines for suspected communicable diseases.

If there is someone unwell on board a flight, the pilot of the aircraft is legally required to inform air traffic control. Arrangements will be made for medical assessments for the person on arrival. The exact arrangements will depend on the airport involved. The local Public Health Team would be alerted if there was a possibility that the individual was suffering from an infectious disease so that appropriate public health action could be initiated.

If we get a case of Ebola in the UK, would we see an outbreak similar to West Africa?

While the UK might see cases of imported Ebola, this is extremely unlikely to result in a large outbreak in the UK. England has a world-class healthcare system with robust infection control systems and processes and disease control systems that have a proven record of dealing with imported infectious diseases.

Is there a risk of Ebola transmission from illegal bushmeat?

The risk to the UK population of acquiring Ebola virus from bushmeat is very low.

It is illegal to import bushmeat into the UK. Cooking will kill the virus, but there is some risk in handling raw bushmeat and the Food Standards Agency advice has always been that people should avoid illegal bushmeat as you can never be certain of its safety.

Why are there media reports of people in the UK being tested for Ebola?

Public Health England has advised frontline medical practitioners to be alert to Ebola in those returning from affected areas. An increase in testing following such advice is to be expected.

To date all those tested have been negative. The initial symptoms of Ebola are similar to a number of other far more common diseases such as malaria and dengue fever.

26 August 2014

⇨ The above information is reprinted with kind permission from NHS Choices. Please visit www.nhs.uk for further information.

© *NHS Choices 2014*

What are vectors?

Vectors are living organisms that can transmit infectious diseases between humans or from animals to humans. Many of these vectors are bloodsucking insects that ingest disease-producing micro-organisms during a blood meal from an infected host (human or animal) and later inject them into a new host during their next blood meal. Mosquitoes are the best known disease vector. Others include certain species of ticks, flies, sandflies, fleas, bugs and freshwater snails.

More than half the world at risk

Vector-borne diseases are illnesses caused by pathogens and parasites in human populations. Every year more than one billion people are infected and more than one million people die from vector-borne diseases including malaria, dengue, schistosomiasis, leishmaniasis, Chagas disease, yellow fever, lymphatic filariasis and onchocerciasis.

One sixth of the illness and disability suffered worldwide is due to vector-borne diseases, with more than half the world's population currently estimated to be at risk of these diseases. The poorest segments of society and least-developed countries are most affected.

These diseases affect urban, peri-urban and rural communities but thrive predominantly among communities with poor living conditions – particularly lack of access to adequate housing, safe drinking water and sanitation. Malnourished people and those with weakened immunity are especially vulnerable.

These diseases also exacerbate poverty. Illness and disability prevent people from working and supporting themselves and their family, causing further hardship and impeding economic development. Dengue, for example, imposes a substantial economic burden on families and governments, both in medical costs and in working days lost due to illness. According to studies from eight countries, an average dengue episode represents 14.8 lost days for ambulatory patients at an average cost of US$514 and 18.9 days for non-fatal hospitalised patients at an average cost of US$1491.

Vector-borne diseases therefore play a central role in poverty reduction and economic development. An econometric model for malaria suggests that countries with intensive malaria have income levels of only one third of those that do not have malaria.

Increasing threat

Back in the 1940s, the discovery of synthetic insecticides was a major breakthrough in the control of vector-borne diseases. Large-scale indoor spraying programmes during the 1950s and 1960s succeeded in bringing many of the major vector-borne diseases under control. By the late 1960s, many of these diseases – with the exception of malaria in Africa – were no longer considered to be of primary public health importance.

This triggered a major setback. Control programmes lapsed, resources dwindled, and specialists in vector control disappeared from public health units.

Within the past two decades, many important vector-borne diseases have re-emerged or spread to new parts of the world. Traditionally regarded as a problem for countries in tropical settings, vector-borne diseases pose an increasingly wider threat to global public health, both in terms of the number of people affected and their geographical spread.

Their potential to spread globally, changes in climate, ecology, land-use patterns, and the rapid and increased movement of people and goods is threatening more than half the world's population.

Environmental changes are causing an increase in the number and spread of many vectors worldwide. Dengue in particular is emerging as a serious public health concern. In 2012, it ranked as the most important mosquito-borne viral disease with epidemic potential in the world. There has been a 30-fold increase in cases during the past 50 years, and its human and economic costs are staggering.

The primary vector for dengue, the *Aedes aegypti* mosquito, is now found in more than 20 European countries. This same mosquito species recently carried chikungunya to the Caribbean islands; the first cases of this debilitating disease seen in the Region of the Americas.

Alongside this alarming spread of vectors is the serious concern of increasing insecticide resistance. Today most species of vectors are showing resistance to many classes of insecticides. If existing insecticides lose their effectiveness this could erase all the gains made against malaria and other vector-borne diseases, especially in parts of Africa.

And at the same time, the world is facing an extreme shortage of entomologists and vector-control experts. Very few African countries have entomologists and vector-control experts. Very few African countries have entomology programmes at undergraduate university level and some countries have only a handful of expert entomologists.

2014

⇨ The above information is reprinted with kind permission from the World Health Organization. Please visit www.who.int for further information.

Vectors and the diseases that they can transmit	
Vector	**Diseases**
Mosquitos	
Aedes aegypti	Dengue, yellow fever, chikungunya, Zika virus
Aedes albopictus	Chikungunya, dengue, West Nile virus
Culex quinquefasciatus	Lymphatic filariasis
Anopheles (more than 60 known species can transmit diseases)	Malaria, lymphatic filariasis (in Africa)
Haemagogus	Yellow fever
Sandflies	Leishmaniasis
Triatomine bugs	Chagas disease
Ticks	Crimean-Congo haemorrhagic fever, tick-borne encephalitis, typhus, Lyme disease
Fleas	Plague, Murine typhus
Flies (various species)	Human African trypanosomiasis, onchocerciasis

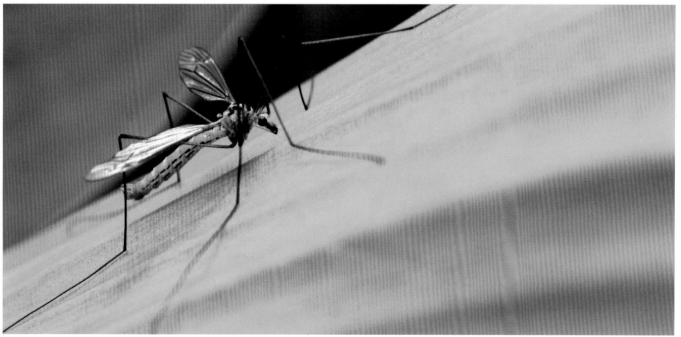

Malaria maps reveal that 184 million Africans still live in extremely high-risk areas despite decade of control efforts

40 African countries showed reductions in malaria transmission between 2000–2010, but despite this progress, more than half (57 per cent) of the population in countries endemic for malaria continue to live in areas of moderate to intense transmission, with infection rates over ten per cent. The findings are based on a series of prevalence maps for malaria published this week in The Lancet.

A team led by Dr Abdisalan Noor and Professor Robert Snow of the KEMRI-Wellcome Trust Research Programme produced the maps by geocoding data from surveys in 44 African countries and territories endemic for malaria in order to identify which populations were at risk of the disease in 2000 and 2010.

The time period coincides with the launch of the Roll Back Malaria Partnership, which brought with it a large increase in investment targeting malaria control, and the team aimed to investigate the progress in reducing transmission during this period. Their maps revealed that the number of people living in high-risk areas, where more than 50 per cent of the population are likely to carry infections, fell from 219 million in 2000 to 184 million in 2010, a fall of 16 per cent.

However, the maps also identified that just ten countries harbour 87 per cent of the population remaining at high-risk of disease transmission, and intensity remained high or unchanged in eight countries including the Democratic Republic of Congo, Uganda, Malawi and South Sudan.

To ensure accuracy, the study used measurements for the prevalence of malaria in populations where diagnosis had been confirmed through laboratory techniques.

'Health information systems in many African countries are weak and it has been difficult to reliably estimate how many people get sick, or die, of malaria,' said Dr Abdisalan, Noor, who led the study. 'The population surveys we used in this study are a more reliable indicator for tracking and we hope our study will help countries assess their progress and adapt their strategies for more effective malaria control.'

The study is one of the largest examples of mapping and modelling for any parasitic disease in Africa and is the first study to look at the changing intensity of malaria transmission across the African continent in order to assess the impact from the first ten years of the Roll Back Malaria Partnership.

Professor Robert Snow, who co-authored the study,

said: 'The results of our analysis are pause for thought. On the one hand it's a glass half full, with several countries showing significant reductions in malaria transmission, and on the other it's a glass half empty, where, despite a decade of massive investment in malaria control the populations living in several African countries are as likely to be infected with malaria in 2000 as they were ten years later.'

Dr Noor added: 'Advanced skills in spatial statistics and computing are enabling us to measure changes in malaria transmission in new ways and where they are most needed. By continuing to bring together dedicated scientists in Africa we can have better monitoring and tailor control of malaria transmission in the future.'

Despite the reductions seen the paper highlights the need for global support to sustain and further accelerate a decrease in malaria transmission.

The project was a pan-African effort using data provided by national malaria control programmes, researchers in sub-Saharan Africa and national and international archives.

21 February 2014

⇨ The above information is reprinted with kind permission from the Wellcome Trust. Please visit www.wellcome.ac.uk for further information.

© *Wellcome Trust 2014*

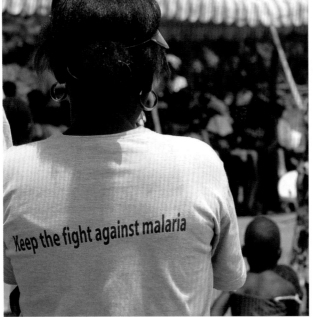

Keep the fight against malaria

Non-communicable diseases (NCDs): a global emergency

NCDs – a fast growing epidemic.

⇨ NCDs kill 36 million people a year – more than all other causes combined. They are the most frequent cause of death in most countries and account for nearly two thirds of all deaths globally.

⇨ If current trends continue, NCD deaths will increase by 15 per cent over the next decade, reaching 44 million a year.

⇨ While infectious disease deaths are projected to decline by about seven million over the next 20 years, cardiovascular disease and cancer deaths are expected to increase by ten million.

⇨ The World Economic Forum identifies NCDs as a top threat to the global economy.

NCDs hit low- and middle-income countries hardest

⇨ Nearly four out of five deaths (80%) from NCDs occur in low- or middle-income countries.

⇨ If current trends continue, by 2030 NCDs in low- and middle-income countries will cause FIVE times more deaths than communicable diseases, maternal and newborn death and hunger combined.

⇨ NCDs kill people at a younger age in low- and middle-income countries – on average ten years younger than in high-income countries.

⇨ While Africa is the one region where communicable diseases still kill more people than NCDs, even there NCDs are rising fast and it is expected that by 2030 the toll of NCDs will nearly equal the toll of communicable disease, maternal and newborn death and malnutrition combined.

⇨ In a single decade, developing countries are expected to lose 84 billion dollars of productivity from the death and disability caused by NCDs.

NCDs can be prevented

⇨ A large percentage of NCDs can be prevented by reducing the four main shared risk factors: tobacco use, physical inactivity, harmful use of alcohol and unhealthy diet.

⇨ At least 80 per cent of premature heart disease, stroke and type 2 diabetes can be prevented.

We must take action now to:

⇨ Target whole populations with a comprehensive approach that includes both prevention and treatment of NCDs.

⇨ In low-resource settings, ensure that cost-effective interventions ('best buys') are given highest priority (e.g. implementation of the Framework Convention on Tobacco Control, restrictions on use of alcohol, reduction of salt intake, replacement of trans-fats, mass media promotion of physical activity).

⇨ Find out about risk factors in your country and influence policymakers to take measures to reduce the factors that affect your population most.

⇨ Develop collaboration between governments, international agencies, civil society actors and the private sector to work together to adopt cost-effective measures that counter these threats.

⇨ Join forces through the NCD Alliance and urge governments to make concrete commitments at the UN High-level Meeting on NCDs and beyond.

What are NCDs, and what causes them?

Non-communicable diseases include: cancer, cardiovascular disease, chronic respiratory disease and diabetes. Tobacco use, unhealthy diet and physical inactivity are responsible for the vast majority of death and disability caused by NCDs. These threats have increased dramatically with recent global changes such as

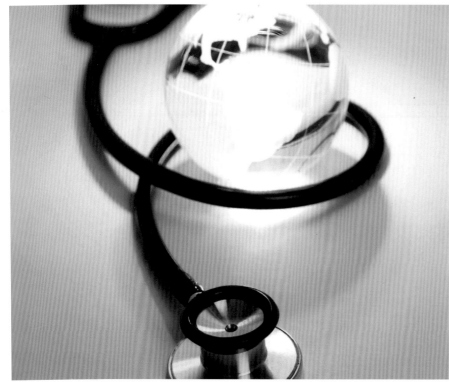

globalisation and urbanisation, and related demographic, economic and technological developments. Urbanisation, employment patterns, social trends and mass communication work together to create an environment that restricts choices and shapes the behaviours that influence health, including quality of diet and level of physical activity. In extremely low-income countries, many NCDs are linked to infections. These include rheumatic heart disease, cervical cancer, liver cancer and stomach cancer.

Why are the poor more vulnerable to NCDs?

NCDs affect men, women and children of all social and economic levels. The large majority of those suffering from NCDs live in low- and middle-income countries. In high-income settings, NCDs are most common among the poor. Poverty is both a cause and a consequence of NCDs. Limited access to healthcare, insurance and/or social benefits in low-income countries means that the death or disability of a breadwinner often impoverishes an extended family. The loss of productivity of workers killed or disabled by NCDs is enormous and it threatens to undermine the economic growth of many developing and emerging economies. NCDs impede progress toward the Millennium Development Goals, especially those on factors affecting health like poverty and education.

Why are NCDs neglected in low- and middle-income countries?

Many people still believe that NCDs primarily affect the wealthy. NCDs are seldom seen to be a health priority in low- and middle-income countries. Because the behaviours that contribute so heavily to NCD risk are shaped by policy, norms and environmental factors, solutions require the commitment and collaboration of many sectors that are not accustomed to taking health needs into account.

What can be done?

Governments, civil society and elements of the private sector are beginning to recognise that we must invest in NCD prevention to protect socio-economic development. Policymakers, educators, healthcare providers, corporations, municipal authorities, the media and others are starting to work together to raise the priority given to non-communicable diseases, to increase resources allotted to them and to move people to action. Effective tobacco control policies, changes in food content, guidelines and policy on labelling and marketing, plus city planning that facilitates active (as opposed to motorised) transport are among the measures that will help get the NCD epidemic under control.

⇨ The above information is reprinted with kind permission from the World Heart Federation. Please visit www.world-heart-federation.org for further information.

© World Heart Federation 2014

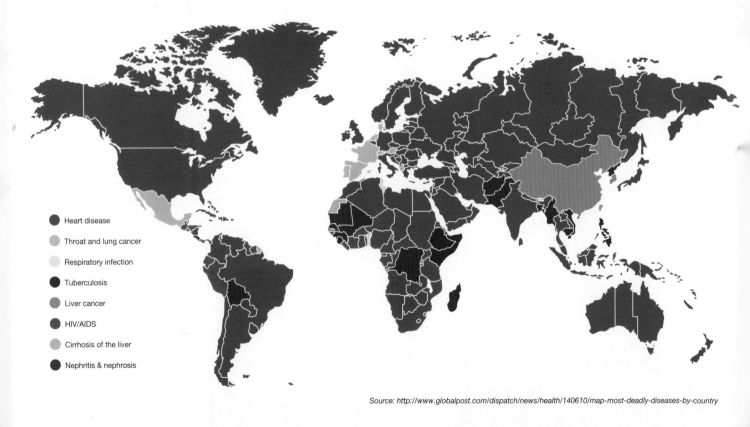

What diseases do people die of in different parts of the world?

- Heart disease
- Throat and lung cancer
- Respiratory infection
- Tuberculosis
- Liver cancer
- HIV/AIDS
- Cirrhosis of the liver
- Nephritis & nephrosis

Source: http://www.globalpost.com/dispatch/news/health/140610/map-most-deadly-diseases-by-country

First Hendra, now bat lyssavirus, so what are zoonotic diseases?

An article from The Conversation.

By Linfa Wang, Office of the Chief Executive Science Leader in Virology at CSIRO and Gary Crameri, Virologist, Australian Animal Health Laboratory at CSIRO

The last 30 years have seen a rise in emerging infectious diseases in humans, of which more than 70% are zoonotic. Zoonoses are diseases that normally exist in animals but have the potential to transmit to humans. They can be caused by many different infectious agents including bacteria, fungi and viruses.

Zoonotic infections have always been a part of the human disease landscape and most have come from domestic animals. The long lists includes anthrax, tuberculosis, plague, yellow fever and influenza. But with changes in environment, human behaviour and habitat destruction, these biosecurity threats are increasingly emerging from wildlife species.

Although it was established over a century ago that rabies was linked to bats, the research community was surprised to find that the SARS virus – which claimed more than 800 lives and cost more than $80 billion globally – emerged from bats to civets and ultimately infected humans in the wet markets of southern China.

The World Health Organization (WHO) and most infectious disease experts agree that the source of the next human pandemic is likely to be zoonotic and wildlife is likely the prime suspect. While much effort has understandably gone into preparations for avian influenza, the next deadly pandemic may be the result of a currently unknown zoonotic agent.

Since the identification of bats as the probable source of the SARS epidemic, the global focus on emerging infectious disease has turned to them to understand and ultimately predict the source of the next human pandemic.

In the last 20 years, a significant number of highly lethal viral diseases have emerged from bat species across the world. These include Hendra virus and Australian bat lyssavirus in Australia and Nipah virus in Malaysia and Bangladesh, where regular outbreaks reach mortality levels of 100%. Haemorrhagic fever viruses, including the feared and lethal Ebola and Marburg viruses, have also emerged from bats in Africa and Asia.

After crippling the globe in 2003 and 2004, SARS appeared to have vanished until last year when there was a deadly human SARS-like outbreak in Saudi Arabia. It killed six out of 12 infected patients and cases of infection continue to emerge. Known as SARI (severe acute respiratory infection), this infection has now shown the critical capacity to transmit from one person to another and, like its precursor, initial evidence supports its emergence from bats.

Zoonotic diseases in humans can take several different courses. For some, like rabies and West Nile virus, humans are 'dead-end' hosts. That is, they transmit (spill over) from their animal reservoir (host) into humans but as there's no subsequent human-to-human transmission, the disease is restricted from spreading.

Others, such as SARS and avian influenza, spill over to humans, cause disease and are able to transmit from person to person before being eradicated or 'burning out' from the human population, leaving no residual infection except in its animal host.

The third are diseases such as HIV AIDS, which spilled out of primates decades ago and has persisted in the human population ever since. And measles and mumps, which probably entered the human population thousands of years ago and are somewhat controlled but still circulating.

It's impossible to completely safeguard against zoonotic diseases but steps can and are being taken to limit the opportunity for spill-over events through monitoring and rapid response when and where they do occur.

Controlling zoonotic diseases and protecting our animals, people and environment from increasing biosecurity threats will not only take a global effort but a multidisciplinary one. It cannot be addressed adequately with traditional human medical strategies where disease is fought in the human population only.

If we are to prepare and respond adequately to the next zoonotic attack, the approach needs to be diverse, taking in medical, veterinary, ecological and environmental factors. The transition will be complex, but necessary if we are to protect the global community from zoonotic disease as best as we can. After all, the stakes are high.

26 February 2013

Cholera

Cholera often breaks out when there is overcrowding and inadequate access to clean water, rubbish collection and proper toilets. It causes profuse diarrhoea and vomiting which can lead to death by intense dehydration, sometimes within a matter of hours.

Cholera is a serious risk in the aftermath of emergencies, like the Haiti earthquake of 2010, but can strike anywhere. The situation can be especially problematic in rainy seasons when houses and latrines flood and contaminated water collects in stagnant pools.

According to the World Health Organization (WHO), cholera affects three to five million people worldwide and causes between 100,000 and 130,000 deaths per year.

Médecins Sans Frontières/Doctors Without Borders (MSF)'s water and sanitation engineers and logisticians play a vital role in the prevention of cholera. The disease is treatable and, in many situations, MSF teams have limited the death rate to less than one per cent.

What causes cholera?

Cholera is caused by an infection of the intestine with the bacterium *Vibrio cholerae*. The bacterium causes the cells lining the intestine to produce large amounts of fluid, leading to profuse diarrhoea and vomiting.

The infection spreads when someone ingests food or water contaminated with the faeces or vomit of someone carrying the disease.

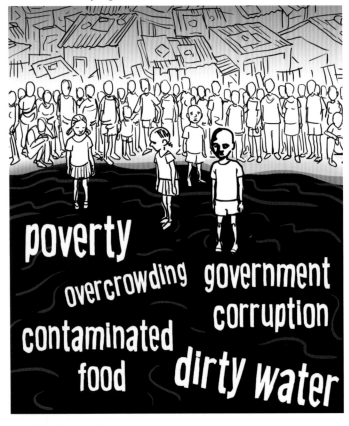

Contaminated food or water supplies can cause massive outbreaks in a short period of time, particularly in overcrowded areas such as slums or refugee camps.

Symptoms of cholera

Typically, symptoms of cholera appear within two to three days of infection. However, it can take anywhere from a few hours to five days or longer for symptoms to appear.

A cholera infection is often mild or without symptoms but can sometimes be severe, resulting in profuse watery diarrhoea, vomiting and leg cramps.

The patient rapidly loses body fluids, leading to dehydration and shock. Without treatment, they may die within hours.

Diagnosing cholera

Cholera can be diagnosed by examining stool samples or rectal swabs but, due to the fast-acting nature of the disease there is often little time to do so.

In epidemic situations, a diagnosis is often made by taking a patient history and conducting a brief examination, with treatment given before there is time for a laboratory to confirm the diagnosis.

Treating cholera

Cholera can be treated simply and successfully by immediately replacing the fluids and salts lost through vomiting and diarrhoea – with prompt rehydration, less than one per cent of cholera patients die.

Cholera victims are always treated with oral rehydration solutions – prepackaged mixtures of sugars and salts that are mixed with water and drunk in large amounts. Severe cases will need these fluids to be replaced intravenously via a drip, and antibiotics are sometimes administered.

2 May 2013

⇨ The above information is reprinted with kind permission from MSF UK. Please visit www.msf.org.uk for further information.

Global health policy fails to address burden of disease on men

Men experience a higher burden of disease and lower life expectancy than women, but policies focusing on the health needs of men are notably absent from the strategies of global health organisations, according to a Viewpoint article in this week's *Lancet*.

The article reinterprets data from the *Global Burden of Disease: 2010* study which shows that all of the top ten causes of premature death and disability, and the top ten behavioural risk factors driving rates of ill-health around the world, affect men more than they affect women.

'Drinking alcohol and smoking are subject to social pressures which have resulted in men globally running three times the risk of ill-health from these behaviours compared to women... We recognise that women are disadvantaged in many societies and consider the advancement of women central to sustainable development, but this does not imply that the international community has no responsibility for men's health too.'

Dr Sarah Hawkes, UCL Institute for Global Health

In every region of the world men die at a younger age than women and the smallest decline in global mortality rates over the past 40 years has been experienced by young men aged 25–39 years.

The commentary, written by Dr Sarah Hawkes of the UCL Institute

for Global Health and Dr Kent Buse of UNAIDS, reviews the responses of major global health institutions and finds that efforts and resources are focussed more often on the health needs of women. The authors argue that global health institutions should start tackling the social norms and commercial interests that push men to take risks with their health.

'Gender norms drive risk-taking,' says Dr Sarah Hawkes. 'Drinking alcohol and smoking, in particular, are subject to social pressures which have resulted in men globally running three times the risk of ill-health from these behaviours compared to women. These norms and customs are clearly perpetuated by all of us, and exploited by commercial interests.'

Dr Hawkes, an expert in sexual health, continues: 'The global health community has made real strides in acknowledging and addressing unsafe sex, we must now do the same for "unsafe gender".

'We recognise that women are disadvantaged in many societies and consider the advancement of women central to sustainable development, but this does not imply that the international community has no responsibility to promote and protect men's health too.'

Co-author Dr Kent Buse, Chief, Political Affairs and Strategy at UNAIDS, says: 'It is more or less universally acknowledged that gender plays a significant role in the risks associated with unsafe/unprotected sex – in this case placing women at greater risk. So why is it so difficult to accept that gender also plays a role in the risk of other major burdens of illness and premature death globally

– particularly those that affect men disproportionately?

'The global health community is taking a short-sighted view,' continues Dr Buse. 'The drivers of ill-health in men are the same drivers of the emerging burden of illness in women. It is time that policy-makers face up to gender in global health and tackle the interests that stand between us and good health for everyone.'

The views were echoed by Professor Chris Murray of the University of Washington, author of the original study on which this analysis is based: 'We as a society should not have lower aspirations for health for males than females. Everyone deserves a chance at a long life in full health, regardless of where they live, their gender or their economic situation.'

Professor Davidson Gwatkin from the Johns Hopkins Bloomberg School of Public Health stated: 'This is by far the most interesting and thought-provoking piece on gender inequalities I have read in a long time. The international health community stands to benefit greatly from such iconoclastic thinking and from the extensive discussion it deserves to generate.'

17 May 2013

⇨ The above information is reprinted with kind permission from UCL. Please visit www.ucl.ac.uk for further information.

New analysis shows current picture of diseases which were widespread in the Victorian era

Hospital admissions for gout increasing, with variation across the country.

New figures published for the first time today paint a current picture of hospital admissions for some diseases that were widespread during the 19th and early 20th centuries.

Hospital admissions for gout are increasing and are highest in patients aged 60 and above, the figures from the Health and Social Care Information Centre (HSCIC) show.

The report is part of the latest monthly provisional Hospital Episode Statistics (HES) publication and also focusses on tuberculosis (TB), whooping cough, measles and malnutrition. It shows that between May 2013 and April 2014:

⇨ Gout admissions have increased by a fifth since 2009-10 in England, with almost 5,800 admissions in the 12 months to April 2014. The latest gout admissions figure is a four per cent rise on the previous 12-month period (5,560) and a 22 per cent rise since 2009–10 (4,760).

⇨ Seven in ten gout admissions were for patients aged 60 and above (4,060 or 70 per cent), with males making up two thirds (2,680 or 66 per cent of this figure).

⇨ There were 86,870 hospital admissions where gout was a primary or secondary diagnosis, an increase of 16 per cent from the same period in 2012–13 (74,960) and an increase of 78 per cent on the same period in 2009–10 (48,720).

Regionally, there was variation for gout and TB admissions by area of residence. Greater Manchester had the highest rate of gout admissions (15.0 per 100,000 population) and

Thames Valley had the lowest (7.9 per 100,000 population). London had the highest rate of TB admissions (15.3 per 100,000 population), with North Yorkshire and the Humber having the lowest (1.5 per 100,000 population).

Admissions also showed variation by deprivation. There were 13.5 gout admissions and 16.5 TB admissions per 100,000 population in the ten per cent most deprived areas, with 8.3 gout admissions and 1.4 TB admissions per 100,000 population in the ten per cent least deprived areas.

Today's report also shows that overall admissions where malnutrition was a primary diagnosis decreased from 683 in 2012–13 to 612 in 2013–14. However, during the same period there was an increase in overall admissions where malnutrition was a primary or secondary diagnosis, from 5,590 to 6,690.

Over the last five years there was a 71 per cent increase in hospital admissions where malnutrition was a primary or secondary diagnosis, from 3,900 admissions in 2009–10 to 6,690 admissions in 2013–14.

The report also showed that the highest mean length of stay in hospital was for malnutrition, at 19.5 days, followed by TB at 13.6 days, gout at 5.2 days and measles at 2.9 days. The lowest mean length of stay was for whooping cough at 2.7 days.

Kingsley Manning, Chair of the HSCIC, said: 'It is fascinating to look at current statistics for some of the diseases and conditions that were prevalent in the 1800s

and early 1900s.

'We are fortunate that these diseases are not as widespread today; however, our figures do show that hospital admissions for gout are increasing. Healthcare organisations may be interested in undertaking further study into the trends highlighted in our report.'

23 July 2014

⇨ The above information is reprinted with kind permission from the Health & Social Care Information Centre. Please visit www.hscic.gov.uk for further information.

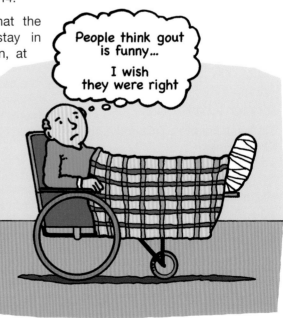

People think gout is funny...

I wish they were right

The influence of westernisation spells danger for public health in Nigeria

Researchers at Warwick Medical School believe that the lifestyle altering effects of westernisation could be responsible for the high prevalence of obesity, and associated health risks, in sub-Saharan Africa.

The study, published in *PLOS ONE*, found that over one in five women in Nigeria were reported to be overweight or obese, with this statistic increasing among demographics with improved social and economic indicators.

Those women classed as having a higher wealth index were three and a half times more likely to be overweight or obese when compared to those in the lowest wealth bracket. Access to higher levels of education also increased risk, as did urbanisation; 36.4% of women in urban areas were overweight compared with 18.8% in more rural districts.

'Obesity is now not just a western problem, but an African one as well,' argues Dr Ngianga-Bakwin Kandala. 'By becoming wealthier, better educated and urbanised regions of Nigeria are gaining the attributes we would more commonly associate with western societies. This has brought both a change in lifestyle and diet that is reflected in finding that educated, wealthy women are much more likely to be obese than those living in more rural, traditional areas.'

'Obesity is now not just a western problem, but an African one as well'

Professor Saverio Stranges explained, 'Urbanisation, and the shift towards what we would consider to be more western habits, appears to come hand in hand with a more sedentary lifestyle and change in diet. More people have cars and drive where they might have walked in the past. The rise in Internet usage within the cities sees more people sat down for prolonged periods, both at home and at work.'

'This physical inactivity is worsened by a less balanced diet. An over- reliance on energy dense processed foods can be highlighted by the growing presence of fast food outlets and the knock-on effect is reducing the intake of staple, low calorie foods.'

This, alongside data from several other countries, suggests that rising urbanisation and improvements in developmental indicators leads to concurrent under- and overnutrition in the population.

This stands to be a continuing problem. In 1995, only 35% of the African population resided in urban areas, a figure projected to rise to 54% by 2030.

Professor Stranges continued, 'The worry is that Nigeria, like many Sub-Saharan African countries, is facing a major public health challenge with a rising number of overweight adults, whilst large segments of the population face problems associated with undernutrition. This dual burden will mean combating both malnutrition and the risks associated with obesity, such as cardiovascular disease.'

'Urbanisation, and the shift towards what we would consider to be more western habits, appears to come hand in hand with a more sedentary lifestyle and change in diet'

Most epidemiological research in sub-Saharan Africa has focused on under-nutrition, particularly within women and children who are deemed to be in the more vulnerable demographics of the population. This new study reflects a growing trend to look at other nutrition problems, and is the first of its kind to do so down to a state level.

The study used data from the 2008 Nigerian Demographic and Health Survey. Around 28,000 women aged between 15 and 49 years old were sampled, of which 20.9% were recorded as being overweight or obese.

Dr Ngianga-Bakwin Kandala added, 'Using such a vast representative population sample we are able to paint a more accurate picture of variances between the individual states for the first time. Lagos State, home to one of the fastest growing cities in the world, reported that over 50% of the women were overweight or obese, whereas the more rural Yobe State in the North East was closer to just 10%.'

'Seeing this data broken down across the states will help to understand both the social and economic burden of obesity, and the future demand upon public health in each state.'

When taking urbanisation and other risk factors into account, the South Eastern states of Cross River, Akwa Ibom, Rivers, Bayelsa and Taraba were shown to have the most significant spatial correlation to being overweight or obese.

With the exception of Kebbi State, those in the north and west had a markedly lower correlation with obesity.

1 July 2014

⇨ The above information is reprinted with kind permission from the University of Warwick. Please visit www.warwick.ac.uk for further information.

Obesity: Africa's new crisis

The arrival of fast food has triggered the latest health epidemic to hit developing countries. As doctors begin the fight back against morbid obesity, Bénédicte Desrus travels round Africa photographing people living with the condition, while Ian Birrell reveals why South Africa now faces its biggest challenge since HIV.

By Ian Birrell

When the first McDonald's restaurant opened almost two decades ago in Johannesburg, a teenage boy named Thando Tshabalala was among the thousands who stood in line patiently waiting to try one of those famous burgers. 'We had seen this place in every movie we ever watched, and it seemed to be mentioned in every song, so I had to try it for myself,' he said.

Given such enthusiasm, it was hardly surprising that South Africa proved to be fertile territory for the burger chain, breaking expansion records with 30 outlets opening in under two years. Today the company operates more than 200 restaurants across the country. When arch-rival Burger King finally entered the market last year it was greeted with similar excitable scenes – almost 5,000 people descended on its launch branch in Cape Town, some even sleeping on the street to ensure they got their hands on a Whopper. 'We did not expect the demand to be so great,' its chairman confessed later.

Tshabalala, now a successful 33-year-old corporate trainer, still enjoys fast food. When we met he was eating a steak sandwich in the food court of a smart shopping mall, sitting among scores of shoppers and families feasting on curries, pizzas, fried fish and the ubiquitous chips. But that skinny teenager has grown into a 5'5" man weighing almost 17 stone – and today he struggles to find clothes to fit his inflated body and complains that seats are becoming too small for comfort.

'To be honest I feel rather self-conscious about my size,' Tshabalala told me with a rueful smile. 'There is this saying in South Africa that if you have a one-pack belly, like a beer belly, you must have lots of money, but if you have a six-pack there is something wrong. But I know it is not really a sign of success to have a big belly.'

Sitting with him was his girlfriend Fiona Sefara, an entrepreneur building a recycling business. A former vegetarian, she recalled leaving South Africa before the end of apartheid to live in America. 'When I went there I was surprised to see all these overweight people on the streets – but when I came back home, McDonald's was everywhere and there were all these bigger people on our own streets.'

As we chatted, she chided her partner for his fondness for fried food and huge portions, then confided that the worst aspect of the change in her homeland was seeing so many overweight children. 'We had nothing as children so we'd take a tennis ball outside and play for hours until it was dark. But now they have computers and are driven everywhere,' she said. 'My own nephew is so chubby that he has become one of those American kids.'

Fat is no longer just a developed world problem. Forget those tired old clichés beloved by the aid industry. Today more people in poorer countries go to bed each night having consumed too many calories than go to bed hungry – a revelation that underlines the breakneck pace of change on our planet. A landmark report by the Overseas Development Institute earlier this year showed that more than one-third of the world's adults are overweight – and that almost two-thirds of the world's overweight people are found in low- and middle-income nations.

The number of obese or overweight people in developing countries rose from 250 million to almost one billion in under three decades, and these rates are rising significantly faster than in rich nations.

South Africa typifies this alarming new trend, with nearly double the average global obesity rates, and according to another report has become the world's third fattest nation. Nearly two-thirds of the population is overweight and, unlike in the developed world, the problem afflicts more women than men. Incredibly, 69.3% of South African females display unhealthy levels of body fat and more than four in ten are clinically obese (defined as having a BMI higher than 30).

These findings emerged in a *Lancet* study published in May which analysed data over a 33-year span from 188 countries. It found the rise in global obesity rates was 'rapid, substantial and widespread, presenting a major public health epidemic in both the developed and developing world'. More than half the women in Botswana and one in eight Nigerian men are also obese, for example, while Egypt saw one of the fastest rises among women.

Obesity is on the rise in poorer nations even among children; more than a quarter of girls and almost one in five boys in South Africa is overweight. 'These are devastating figures, especially since it is such an expensive disease,' said Professor Tess Van der Merwe, who performs weight-loss surgery and is president of the South African Society for Obesity and Metabolism. 'We cannot afford to spend the next decade debating this issue. The obesity problem in our country is where the HIV epidemic was ten years ago, when we turned a blind eye to the scale of the problem in terms of health economics and became the worst in the world in terms of outcomes.'

Terrifying talk for a nation in transition that provides only rudimentary healthcare for most of its population and where a quarter of citizens still struggle with food security. Experts say such diseases such as cancer, cardiovascular conditions and diabetes will soon overtake HIV and tuberculosis as the biggest causes of death in South Africa.

One man who understands the scale of South Africa's challenge is Aaron Motsaoledi, a 56-year-old doctor from Limpopo and the country's current minister of health. 'It is weird when we are seeing malnutrition co-exist alongside obesity,' he told me. 'I am not only sad but also alarmed, because of my medical training. In the next decade many countries will not be able to afford their health costs, and this definitely includes South Africa.'

Motsaoledi believes the problems fit a global pattern of obesity caused by the rapid shift to urban living combined with increased consumption of western-style diets high in sugar, fat and salt. The problem has worsened in South Africa since it is a nation whose love of meat barbecued on the braai cuts across ethnic boundaries – the two groups hit hardest by obesity are white Afrikaner males and black urban females. On top of this, fears over crime have boosted car culture, with cities designed around US-style shopping malls and fewer children running free in the streets.

'30 years ago black people in South Africa were eating produce from fields that was much healthier, and they were walking big distances,' said Motsaoledi. 'When I was a child pupils would walk 6km to school; some even walked 10km each way. Now life has changed and people do not want to walk anywhere.'

The health minister tries to set an example, dropping a few clothes sizes after cutting down on meat and eating more fish and vegetables. But not all the country's political leaders are so diligent – last year there was a scandal after it was discovered that the premier of one province used her government credit card to spend nearly £3,000 on fast food in her first ten weeks in office at outlets such as KFC and Wimpy. And Motsaoledi complains he is dismissed as a health fanatic while food companies chasing profits ignore his attempts at regulation.

Efforts to grapple with this obesity epidemic show the special problems this global concern causes among poorer people in developing nations. One sunny Monday morning I drove to Soweto to visit Petrus Molefe Park, named after a local hero of the liberation struggle. Two years ago the city council installed an impressive 'green gym' for residents. Sure enough, the first person I met was the perfect promoter for the idea: an unemployed man named Vusi, who told me he spent two hours every day pumping iron after abandoning his unhealthy lifestyle.

Then we were joined by three young women, who confessed this was the first time they had come along in a bid to lose weight. I started talking to Octavia Mphumbude, who was tentatively testing a running machine in her turquoise jeans and black cardigan. 'I won't lie – I like junk food a lot,' said the 25-year-old single mother, who has

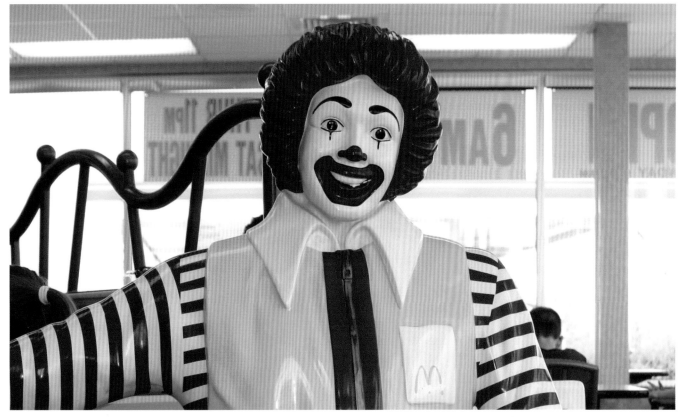

never managed to find a job despite intensive efforts and voluntary work. 'The trouble is, when I am hungry I crave fast food. It is hard to resist. And many of the women around here are unemployed, like me, so if you're unhappy it's comfort food. This is why weight is an issue for us.'

Unfortunately, poor people fill their bellies with cheap food – and this often means salt-drenched starchy carbohydrates, highly processed sweetened products and the fattiest cuts of meat discarded by wealthier consumers. Street-food surveys found that chicken sold in townships is often little more than skin and other meat is just fatty offal, while foreign fast food is seen as sophisticated. Meanwhile mothers go without meals to ensure that their children eat, then gorge when they have money.

All this can lead to 'hidden hunger', when people eat regularly and even put on weight but lack necessary nutrients and vitamins, leading to long-term health damage. 'In one household you can see children who are undernourished, the man with normal weight and then the wife who may be heavily overweight,' said Zandile Mchiza, an expert with the Chronic Diseases of Lifestyle Unit at the Medical Research Council. 'This is why we have the issue of obesity coming up so strongly in Africa even while many people are still starving.'

Mchiza also pointed to cultural issues that fuel obesity in Africa, with big men seen as successful and big women seen as beautiful. 'The majority of black South African men prefer chubby women,' said the 34-year-old scientist. 'If you are too thin it means your husband is not taking care of you or you are unhappy. And your children must be fat, too – we were force fed growing up, always told to eat up all our food and not waste anything on our plates.'

I heard similar claims from other experts – and certainly a glance at the Internet indicates specialist dating sites for 'cuddly' people are booming. A study last year by the Human Sciences Research Council

found that 88% of South Africans regard a fat body as their ideal.

Several township women mentioned told me of another depressing reason not to diet. 'There is a stigma that if you are a black woman and start losing weight you might be ill, you might have HIV,' said Dudu Masooana, a friendly 38-year-old mother of three from Soweto whom I met as she lunched on fried chicken and pap, a traditional porridge made from ground maize. 'This really matters if you are a woman coming from the ghetto.'

A host of parasitical industries have grown up to feed off the obesity crisis, from quack diets and hypnotism at one end of the spectrum to fitness boot camps and bariatric surgery at the other. Television has also got in on the act, with reality shows encouraging people to turn their lives around by exercising and improving diet. One of the most popular is Kabelo's Boot Camp, hosted by a pop star who became a poster boy for healthy living after defeating a drug problem and losing 100lb. Now Kabelo Mabalane runs marathons, eschews substance abuse and puts ten South Africans selected from the thousands of hefty applicants through their paces on his 11-week show.

'We used to associate wealth with a big tummy and had the idea that if you were skinny you were not doing well,' he told me. 'It is only now, 20 years after democracy, that we are dealing with these issues and educating people about the dangers of overeating and obesity. It's a physical transformation, but you have to deal with the issues inside the head, too.'

There are signs that the government recognises the need for action, with the vice president set to lead a commission to bring together academics and officials from different departments to find urgent solutions. The hope is to get the nation to take notice of the crisis; the outlawing of trans fats was ignored by the food industry and the government lacked the ability to police the measure. There has been action taken to reduce salt in

processed foods such as bread and talk of a ban on alcohol advertising, provoking outrage from a powerful industry.

But this is a global crisis. And the surge in South African obesity is simply one more sign that, from Cape Town to Cairo, a continent for too long seen as the poor relation is catching up with the rest of the world as it rapidly grows and urbanises. Obesity is growing faster globally than any other cause of disease. Mexico has rates to match the United States, while the number of overweight people in China – a country that endured horrific famine within living memory – has near-doubled since 1980 as teenagers guzzle fast food and parents shower sweet treats on their solitary children.

There are attempts to grapple with this crisis: restricting trans-fatty acids in Denmark, imposing taxes on fizzy drinks in Mexico, even fines for employers of overweight staff in Japan. But there was one more chilling fact in that recent *Lancet* study looking at three decades of obesity around the world. Not only is one-third of the planet's population too fat – with those numbers rising daily and the problem hitting women especially hard – but perhaps most frighteningly of all, not one of the 188 nations studied managed to reduce obesity levels over the period studied. Truly, as the fast-food joints and shopping malls of South Africa show, this has become a global health and social crisis of gargantuan proportions.

This is an edited version of an article that appeared in *Mosaic: the Science of Life*, a digital publication from the Wellcome Trust (mosaicscience. com).

21 September 2014

⇨ The above information is reprinted with kind permission from *The Guardian*. Please visit www.theguardian.com for further information.

Antimicrobial resistance (AMR): information and resources

Antimicrobial resistance occurs when infections caused by microorganisms no longer respond to treatment.

Antimicrobial resistance is when infections caused by micro-organisms survive exposure to a drug that was supposed to kill them or stop their growth, this is a particular problem with antibiotic resistance. Many of the medical advances in recent years, for example organ transplantation and cancer chemotherapy, need antibiotics to prevent and treat the bacterial infections that can be caused by the treatment. Without effective antibiotics, even minor surgery and routine operations could become high-risk procedures if serious infections can't be treated.

Public Health England (PHE), Department for Environment, Food and Rural Affairs (Defra) and the Department of Health (DH) are leading the implementation of the UK five-year antimicrobial resistance strategy, published in September 2013. A High Level Steering Group has been set up to implement the strategy. The group is working with a range of partners across the human and animal health, research, industry and academic sectors.

Strategic publications

A cross-government UK Five year AMR strategy was published in September 2013.

Public Health England have set up an AMR Strategy Programme Coordination Group to bring together delivery partners from across the health and social care sector. This group will coordinate the implementation of the human health aspects of 4 (out of 7) important areas of the AMRstrategy for England.

'Antimicrobial resistance is when infections caused by micro-organisms survive exposure to a drug that was supposed to kill them or stop their growth'

They have also developed a new national AMR programme; the English Surveillance Programme for Antimicrobial Utilization and Resistance. This programme will monitor the way antibiotics are used by patients and prescribed by doctors across the NHS in England.

14 August 2014

⇨ The above information is reprinted with kind permission from Department of Health, Public Health England and Department for Environment, Food & Rural Affairs. Please visit www.gov.uk for further information.

© Crown copyright 2014

Estimated proportions of multidrug-resistant cases among new and previously treated TN cases, 2012, by WHO region

WHO region	New			Previously treated		
	% MDR	95% confidence intervals		% MDR	95% confidence intervals	
AFR	2.3	0.2	4.4	10.7	4.4	17
AMR	2.2	1.4	3.0	13.5	4.7	22.3
EMR	3.5	0.1	11.3	32.5	11.5	53.5
EUR	15.7	9.5	21.9	45.3	39.2	51.5
SEA	2.2	1.6	2.8	16.1	11.1	21
WPR	4.7	3.3	6.1	22.1	17.6	26.5
Global	3.6	2.1	5.1	20.2	13.3	27.2

AFR: African Region; AMR: Region of Americas; EMR: Eastern Mediterranean Region; EUR: European Region;

MDR: Multidrug resistance; SEA: South-East Asia Region; WPR: Western Pacific Region

Source: Antimicrobial Resistance Global Report on Surveillance, 2014, *World Health Organization*

Study shows why doctors over-prescribe antibiotics

New research from a University of Queensland sociologist shows many doctors over-prescribe antibiotics because they want the best outcomes for individual patients.

University of Queensland Head of Sociology Associate Professor Alex Broom said although health authorities understood the community-wide risks of antibiotic resistance, many doctors were still not complying.

'On any given day in Australia, about 40 per cent of hospital in-patients will receive antibiotics, with between 20 and 50 per cent of those deemed unnecessary or sub-optimal in current best practice terms, depending on the individual hospital,' Associate Professor Broom said.

'Many doctors continue to over-prescribe and mis-prescribe antibiotics, even though they are aware that this can contribute to the proliferation of drug-resistant bacteria.

'There is broad recognition among researchers that in the next few decades there will be no antibiotic options left to treat the rapidly increasing number of highly resistant superbugs, creating the possibility of a global antimicrobial

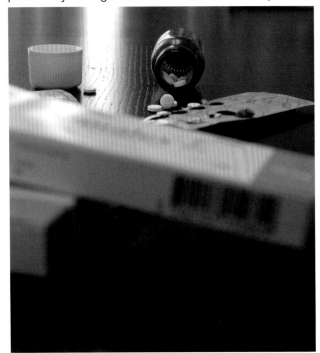

perfect storm,' Associate Professor Broom said..

Associate Professor Broom said attempts to change hospital doctors' use of antibiotics had seen little success.

In a collaborative study between Sunshine Coast Hospital and Health Service Infection Diseases Department and UQ's School of Social Science, 30 hospital-based doctors from a range of specialities were interviewed.

Findings showed that despite understanding the long-term risks of resistance, most doctors still promoted unnecessary use of antibiotics.

'We found that doctors are focussed almost exclusively on treating the potential infection in front of them, in their individual patient,' Associate Professor Broom said.

'Long-term risks are not prioritised and the judicious use of antibiotics is not valued,

'On night shifts, junior staff reported over-prescribing antibiotics to avoid having to wake a senior doctor and ask for help.

'They were also worried about the risk of not acting to prevent or treat the infection.'

Associate Professor Broom said although such actions are rationalised, they were contributing to the global crisis of diminishing effects of many antibiotics and the proliferation of resistant bacteria.

'Overuse by doctors also exposes their patients to unnecessary and sometimes serious drug side-effects of potent antibiotics,' he said.

Associate Professor Broom said strategies to improve antibiotic prescribing practices in hospitals had largely failed because they did not take into account the effects of doctors' abilities to balance immediate risks versus long-term population consequences.

'The immediate perceived professional risks of being seen as under-treating patients were consistently described as hugely outweighing the longer-term population risks of over-treating and thus contributing to resistance,' he said.

'This results in doctors prescribing early rather than adopting a "wait and see" approach.'

The results of this research reveal a major challenge to Australian doctors in terms of whether they are able and willing to prioritise long-term antibiotic protection to ensure the health of Australia's future generations.

'This will likely need to be addressed on multiple levels including within medical training and addressing individual hospital hierarchies and practices that do not confirm with established national guidelines,' Associate Professor Broom said.

28 March 2014

⇨ The above information is reprinted with kind permission from The University of Queensland, Australia. Please visit www.uq.edu.au for further information.

41% of adults think antibiotics kill viruses

Most British adults know when not to use antibiotics, but a sizeable minority have the wrong idea.

By William Jordan

David Cameron recently drew attention to the growing threat of antibiotic resistant strains of bacteria, saying the failure to act could cast the world 'back into the dark ages of medicine'. MPs have also warned that antibiotics have come to be treated as a 'cure-all' and called for new steps to stop doctors and vets from prescribing them when they are not essential. Antibiotics are drugs designed to kill bacteria and not viruses. Drug resistance can develop when antibiotics are given out for conditions they are not designed to treat, such as viral infections, and also when patients suffering from a bacterial infection quit their regimen too soon, before the bacteria is killed off completely.

New YouGov research suggests a significant minority of British adults are misinformed about when it is appropriate to use antibiotics.

In particular, 41% of British adults say a viral infection can usually be 'cured' by taking the wrong antibiotics.

Between 16 and 24% also think antibiotics can usually cure ailments like a cough, the flu or a 'regular' sore throat. While it is true that certain specific coughs and sore throats stemming from bacterial infections (like tonsillitis) can be cured with antibiotics, the NHS does not recommend using, because most coughs and sore throats are caused by viruses.

Another 8% say antibiotics can cure the common cold, which is always caused by a virus.

The survey also found that 7% of adults have used antibiotics when the drugs were not even prescribed by a doctor, and 18% have finished taking antibiotics before the end of a course. If a course is not completed, it is more likely that some bacteria will survive and develop resistance to the drug used.

NHS figures show that the prescription of antibiotic drugs has increased by 30% since the year 2000, and an estimated 5,000 people die each year because of drug-resistant strains of bacteria.

8 July 2014

⇨ The above information is reprinted with kind permission from YouGov. Please visit www.yougov.co.uk for further information.

To the best of your knowledge, which of the following conditions can usually be cured by taking the right antibiotics?

Condition	Can be cured using antibiotics	Can't be cured using antibiotics	Don't know
Bacterial infection	88%	8%	4%
Ear infection	80%	11%	9%
Kidney infection	77%	11%	13%
Pneumonia	70%	16%	14%
Viral infection	41%	54%	5%
regular sore throat	24%	66%	10%
Flu	21%	74%	5%
Common cold	8%	87%	5%
Aches and pains	7%	87%	6%
A hangover	2%	92%	6%

Source: YouGov, July 2014

Seven million premature deaths annually linked to air pollution

In new estimates released today, WHO reports that in 2012 around seven million people died – one in eight of total global deaths – as a result of air pollution exposure. This finding more than doubles previous estimates and confirms that air pollution is now the world's largest single environmental health risk. Reducing air pollution could save millions of lives.

New estimates

In particular, the new data reveal a stronger link between both indoor and outdoor air pollution exposure and cardiovascular diseases, such as strokes and ischaemic heart disease, as well as between air pollution and cancer. This is in addition to air pollution's role in the development of respiratory diseases, including acute respiratory infections and chronic obstructive pulmonary diseases.

The new estimates are not only based on more knowledge about the diseases caused by air pollution, but also upon better assessment of human exposure to air pollutants through the use of improved measurements and technology. This has enabled scientists to make a more detailed analysis of health risks from a wider demographic spread that now includes rural as well as urban areas.

Regionally, low- and middle-income countries in the WHO South-East Asia and Western Pacific Regions had the largest air pollution-related burden in 2012, with a total of 3.3 million deaths linked to indoor air pollution and 2.6 million deaths related to outdoor air pollution.

'Cleaning up the air we breathe prevents noncommunicable diseases as well as reduces disease risks among women and vulnerable groups, including children and the elderly,' says Dr Flavia Bustreo, WHO Assistant Director-General Family, Women and Children's Health. 'Poor women and children pay a heavy price from indoor air pollution since they spend more time at home breathing in smoke and soot from leaky coal and wood cook stoves.'

Included in the assessment is a breakdown of deaths attributed to specific diseases, underlining that the vast majority of air pollution deaths are due to cardiovascular diseases as follows:

Outdoor air pollution-caused deaths – breakdown by disease:

⇨ 40% – ischaemic heart disease;

⇨ 40% – stroke;

⇨ 11% – chronic obstructive pulmonary disease (COPD);

⇨ 6% – lung cancer; and

⇨ 3% – acute lower respiratory infections in children.

Indoor air pollution-caused deaths – breakdown by disease:

⇨ 34% – stroke;

⇨ 26% – ischaemic heart disease;

⇨ 22% – COPD;

⇨ 12% – acute lower respiratory infections in children; and

⇨ 6% – lung cancer.

The new estimates are based on the latest WHO mortality data from 2012 as well as evidence of health risks from air pollution exposures. Estimates of people's exposure to outdoor air pollution in different parts of the world were formulated through a new global data mapping. This incorporated satellite data, ground-level monitoring measurements and data on pollution emissions from key sources, as well as modelling of how pollution drifts in the air.

Risks factors are greater than expected

'The risks from air pollution are now far greater than previously thought or understood, particularly for heart disease and strokes,' says Dr Maria Neira, Director of WHO's Department for Public Health, Environmental and Social Determinants of Health. 'Few risks have a greater impact on global health today than air pollution; the evidence signals the need for concerted action to clean up the air we all breathe.'

After analysing the risk factors and taking into account revisions in methodology, WHO estimates indoor air pollution was linked to 4.3 million deaths in 2012 in households cooking over coal, wood and biomass stoves. The new estimate is explained by better information about pollution exposures among the estimated 2.9 billion people living in homes using wood, coal or dung as their primary cooking fuel, as well as evidence about air pollution's role in the development of cardiovascular and respiratory diseases, and cancers.

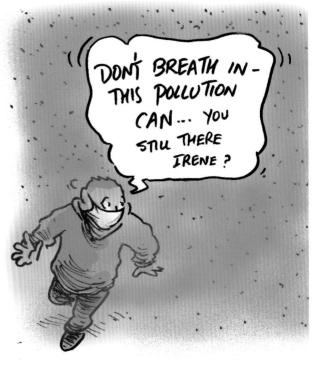

In the case of outdoor air pollution, WHO estimates there were 3.7 million deaths in 2012 from urban and rural sources worldwide.

Many people are exposed to both indoor and outdoor air pollution. Due to this overlap, mortality attributed to the two sources cannot simply be added together, hence the total estimate of around seven million deaths in 2012.

'Excessive air pollution is often a by-product of unsustainable policies in sectors such as transport, energy, waste management and industry. In most cases, healthier strategies will also be more economical in the long term due to healthcare cost savings as well as climate gains,' says Dr Carlos Dora, WHO Coordinator for Public Health, Environmental and Social Determinants of Health. 'WHO and health sectors have a unique role in translating scientific evidence on air pollution into policies that can deliver impact and improvements that will save lives.'

The release of today's data is a significant step in advancing a WHO roadmap for preventing diseases related to air pollution. This involves the development of a WHO-hosted global platform on air quality and health to generate better data on air pollution-related diseases and strengthened support to countries and cities through guidance, information and evidence about health gains from key interventions.

Later this year, WHO will release indoor air quality guidelines on household fuel combustion, as well as country data on outdoor and indoor air pollution exposures and related mortality, plus an update of air quality measurements in 1,600 cities from all regions of the world.

25 March 2014

⇨ The above information is reprinted with kind permission from the World Health Organization. Please visit www.who.int for further information.

Water, sanitation and hygiene

Introduction

According to the latest estimates of the WHO/UNICEF Joint Monitoring Programme for Water Supply and Sanitation (JMP), released in early 2013 (collected in 2011), 36 per cent of the world's population – 2.5 billion people – lack improved sanitation facilities, and 768 million people still use unsafe drinking water sources. Inadequate access to safe water and sanitation services, coupled with poor hygiene practices, kills and sickens thousands of children every day, and leads to impoverishment and diminished opportunities for thousands more.

Poor sanitation, water and hygiene have many other serious repercussions. Children – and particularly girls – are denied their right to education because their schools lack private and decent sanitation facilities. Women are forced to spend large parts of their day fetching water. Poor farmers and wage earners are less productive due to illness, health systems are overwhelmed and national economies suffer. Without WASH (water, sanitation and hygiene), sustainable development is impossible.

UNICEF works in more than 100 countries around the world to improve water supplies and sanitation facilities in schools and communities, and to promote safe hygiene practices. We sponsor a wide range of activities and work with many partners, including families, communities, governments and like-minded organisations. In emergencies we provide urgent relief to communities and nations threatened by disrupted water supplies and disease. All UNICEF WASH programmes were designed to contribute to the Millennium Development Goal for water and sanitation. The goal – to halve, by 2015, the proportion of people without sustainable access to safe water – has been achieved globally, but the same target for sanitation is so far off track that it is unlikely to be met by 2015.

The big picture

Children's rights to an adequate standard of living and to the highest attainable standard of health are enshrined in the Convention on the Rights of the Child. The fulfilment of these rights is the ultimate goal of UNICEF's water, sanitation and hygiene (WASH) programmes.

WASH is a central component of the millennium development agenda. The 2012 update report of the Joint Monitoring Programme for Water Supply and Sanitation (JMP) contained both good and bad news: the Millennium Development Goals (MDGs) drinking water target has been achieved globally, but the sanitation target is so far off track that it is unlikely to be met by 2015. Without significant improvements in sanitation access and hygiene practices, the MDGs related to child mortality, primary education, disease reduction, and poverty eradication will not be achieved.

The MDGs include the specific water and sanitation target of halving, by 2015, the proportion of people without sustainable access to safe drinking water and basic sanitation. According to the latest estimates, the water component of this target was met in 2010. However, 768 million people still lack access to improved drinking water, and the world is not on track to meet the sanitation component. UNICEF is also working to meet a second target of ensuring that all schools have adequate child-friendly water and sanitation facilities and hygiene education programmes. To meet these targets, UNICEF is guided by a new set of strategies that defines the shape of UNICEF WASH programmes to 2015.

UNICEF is part of a growing global effort to meet this challenge. Together with governments, NGOs and other external support agencies, UNICEF is expanding its efforts to meet the WASH challenge.

WASH and health

Poor sanitation, unsafe water and unhygienic practices cause millions of children in the developing world to suffer needlessly from disease. Water- and sanitation-related disease, despite being preventable, remains one of the most significant child health problems worldwide.

Diarrhoea is the most serious of these diseases, alone killing over 3,000 children each day. 88% of diarrhoeal disease is attributed to unsafe drinking water, inadequate sanitation and poor hygiene. Children in developing countries typically have four to five bouts of diarrhoea a year. Even when they don't kill, these diarrhoea episodes can physically and mentally stunt children, affecting them for the rest of their lives. By weakening children, diarrhoea increases mortality rates from other opportunistic diseases, including ARI (acute respiratory infections). ARI and diarrhoea together account for two-thirds of all child deaths worldwide.

Millions of other children are made sick, weakened or are disabled by other water- and sanitation-related diseases and infections including cholera, malaria, trachoma, schistosomiasis, worm infestations and guinea worm disease. And in a growing number of countries, natural or man-made pollution of water sources with dangerous contaminants threatens millions of people.

Access to improved water and sanitation facilities does not, on its own, necessarily lead to improved health. There is now very clear evidence showing the importance of hygienic behaviour, in particular hand-washing with soap at critical times: after defecating and before eating or preparing food. Hand-washing with soap can significantly reduce the incidence of diarrhoea, which is the second leading cause of death amongst children under five years old. In fact, recent studies suggest that regular hand-washing with soap at critical times can reduce the number of diarrhoea bouts by almost 50 per cent.

Good hand-washing practices have also been shown to reduce the incidence of other diseases, notably pneumonia, trachoma, scabies, skin and eye infections and diarrhoea-related diseases like cholera and dysentery. The promotion of hand-washing with soap is also a key strategy for controlling the spread of Avian Influenza (bird flu).

The key to increasing the practice of hand-washing with soap is to promote behavioural change through motivation, information and education. There are a variety of ways to do this including high-profile national media campaigns, peer-to-peer education techniques, hygiene lessons for children in schools and the encouragement of children to demonstrate good hygiene to their families and communities.

It is also true that without water there is no hygiene. Research shows that the less readily available water is, the less likely that good hygiene will be practised in households.

December 2013

⇨ The above information is reprinted with kind permission from UNICEF. Please visit www.unicef.org for further information.

© UNICEF 2014

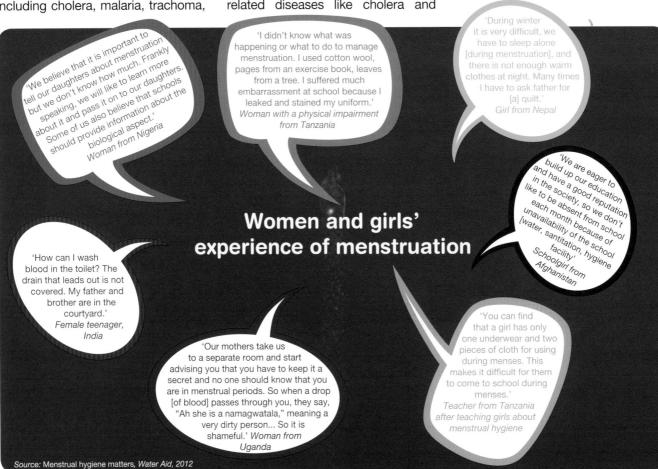

Women and girls' experience of menstruation

'We believe that it is important to tell our daughters about menstruation but we don't know how much. Frankly speaking, we will like to learn more about it and pass it on to our daughters. Some of us also believe that schools should provide information about the biological aspect.'
Woman from Nigeria

'I didn't know what was happening or what to do to manage menstruation. I used cotton wool, pages from an exercise book, leaves from a tree. I suffered much embarrassment at school because I leaked and stained my uniform.'
Woman with a physical impairment from Tanzania

'During winter it is very difficult, we have to sleep alone [during menstruation], and there is not enough warm clothes at night. Many times I have to ask father for [a] quilt.'
Girl from Nepal

'We are eager to build up our education and have a good reputation in the society, so we don't like to be absent from school each month because of unavailability of the school [water, sanitation, hygiene] facility.'
Schoolgirl from Afghanistan

'How can I wash blood in the toilet? The drain that leads out is not covered. My father and brother are in the courtyard.'
Female teenager, India

'Our mothers take us to a separate room and start advising you that you have to keep it a secret and no one should know that you are in menstrual periods. So when a drop [of blood] passes through you, they say, "Ah she is a namagwatala," meaning a very dirty person... So it is shameful.' *Woman from Uganda*

'You can find that a girl has only one underwear and two pieces of cloth for using during menses. This makes it difficult for them to come to school during menses.'
Teacher from Tanzania after teaching girls about menstrual hygiene

Source: Menstrual hygiene matters, Water Aid, 2012

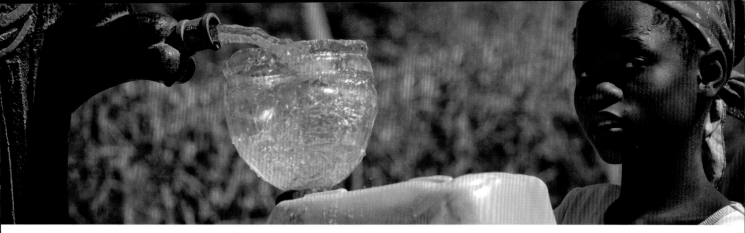

We can't wait

Preface by Gail Klintworth, Chief Sustainability Officer, Unilever

Poor sanitation is an issue that can affect everyone, but women are often the most at risk. As a woman who grew up in a country with sanitation challenges, I was acutely aware of the issues faced by people growing up in rural and evolving urban environments where the infrastructure provided many challenges. I have great empathy with the far-reaching impact this can have on all aspects of a woman's life from childhood through to motherhood and beyond. A lack of access to a clean, safe toilet can impact girls' attendance at school, increase women's burden of work and leave females at risk of sanitation-borne diseases and even violent assault.

The sanitation crisis is an issue which I am passionate about addressing. Improving sanitation would make 1.25 billion women's lives both safer and healthier. Improved sanitation could mean every girl being able to stay in school when she reaches puberty, and all women having a safe place to go so that they are free from fear of assault and the loss of dignity from going in the open. It could free women from the burden of helping their children and family members use a toilet which is far from home and difficult to use. It would help women to take on paid work and to stay at work during menstruation so that they can earn more and invest this back into a better life for themselves and their families. Every day around 2,000 mothers lose a child to diarrhoea caused by lack of access to safe toilets and clean water. I want to see an end to the disease which sanitation brings to women and their families.

At a global level, we simply can't wait to address the sanitation crisis. Of all the Millennium Development Goals, the target to halve the proportion of the global population without sustainable access to safe sanitation is lagging the furthest behind. 2.5 billion people still lack access to toilets. That's more than one in every three people. It's worth stopping to think about that. And this number is likely to increase rather than decrease due to rapid urbanisation unless we take urgent action now.

Executive summary, co-authored by Unilever Domestos, Wateraid and the Water Supply & Sanitation Collaborative Council (WSCC)

There are still 2.5 billion people, or over one third of the world's population, without access to adequate sanitation. Basic sanitation is now recognised as a fundamental human right, the deprivation of which affects the social, physical and economic well-being of societies world-wide.

The challenge of achieving target 7 of the Millennium Development Goals – to halve the proportion of people without sustainable access to safe drinking water and basic sanitation – and MDG 4 – to reduce the under-five mortality rate by two-thirds – could be met by sustained partnerships between governments, businesses, NGOs and communities.

Significant progress has been made towards achieving these targets. Since 1990, almost 1.9 billion more people now have access to improved sanitation. But this is not enough. If progress continues at the current rate the global community will not meet

MDG 7C by 2015. There are still 45 countries in the world where less than half of the population has access to adequate sanitation facilities. Around 700,000 children die every year from diarrhoea caused by unsafe water and poor sanitation. That's almost 2,000 children a day.

Poor sanitation has significant impacts on the safety, well-being and educational prospects of women. Girls' lack of access to a clean, safe toilet, especially during menstruation, perpetuates risk, shame and fear. This has long-term impacts on women's health, education, livelihoods and safety but it also impacts the economy, as failing to provide for the sanitation needs of women ultimately risks excluding half the potential workforce.

Working together, Unilever Domestos, Wateraid and WSSCC recommend that:

⇨ Governments make strengthening the sanitation sector and bringing the MDG target back on track an immediate and urgent political priority.

⇨ Governments (of both developing and donor countries) across the world keep their promises and implement the commitments made at national level, regional level (AfricaSan[1], SACOSAN[2]) and global level (Sanitation and Water

---

1 AfricaSan is a platform created to address the sanitation challenges in Africa. The 5th AfricaSan is scheduled to be held in September 2014. For more information, http://www.amcow-online.org/index.php?option=com_content&view=article&id=71&Itemid=87&lang=en.

2 South Asian Conference on Sanitation (SACOSAN) is a government-led biennial convention held on a rotational basis in each SAARC country and provides a platform for interaction on sanitation. The 5th SACOSAN is being held in Nepal from 22–24 October 2013. For more information, http://www.sacosanv.gov.np/.

for All[3]). Furthermore, they must significantly increase financial resources to the sector, use these resources wisely and ensure that the most marginalised and vulnerable people are targeted.

⇨ The post-2015 development framework must have a clear focus on eradicating extreme poverty by 2030, and UN Member States are urged to consider a dedicated goal on water and sanitation that sets ambitious targets to achieve universal access to water, sanitation and hygiene so that:

- No-one practises open defecation.

- Everyone has safe water, sanitation and hygiene at home.

3 Sanitation and Water for All (SWA) is a partnership of governments, donors, civil society and multilateral organisations. Its aim is to ensure that all people have access to basic sanitation and safe drinking water. For more information, http://www.sanitationandwaterforall.org/.

- All schools and health facilities have safe water, sanitation and hygiene.

- Water, sanitation and hygiene are sustainable and inequalities in access have been progressively eliminated.

⇨ Sanitation should be integrated into education policy supported by sufficient resources and concrete plans to ensure that:

- All schools have adequate sanitation facilities including hand-washing facilities and separate toilets for boys and girls with access for students with disabilities.

- Specific provision is made at school for establishing proper menstrual hygiene management facilities.

- Hygiene promotion is featured as an important part

of the school curriculum from primary level.

⇨ The role for public private partnerships in addressing the sanitation crisis has been formally recognised. More actors in the private sector must realise the social and business opportunities and invest in social development. More frequent and cross-sector collaboration is essential to achieving real progress.

And we must help break the taboo to get the world talking about this urgent and devastating issue, #wecantwait.

⇨ The above information is reprinted with kind permission from WaterAid. Please visit www.wateraid.org for further information.

© WaterAid 2014

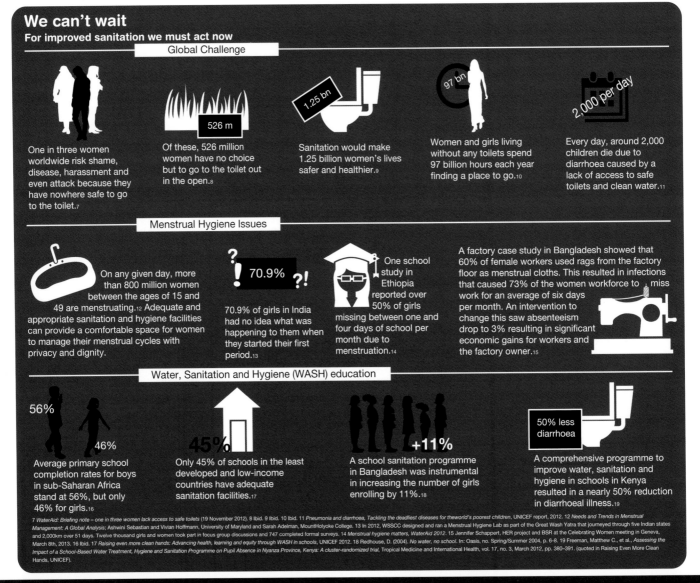

Access to medicines: challenges and opportunities for developing countries

Despite their economic and cultural diversities, the BRICS countries, an association of five major emerging national economies – Brazil, Russian Federation, India, China and South Africa – are facing similar healthcare challenges, including access to health services and medicines, growing health costs, infectious diseases, such as HIV and tuberculosis, and the growing prevalence of non-communicable diseases.

In order to find solutions on how to provide health care to millions of people, in particular the most vulnerable, representatives from BRICS and other low- and middle-income countries met on 19 May in Geneva, on the sidelines of the 67th World Health Assembly.

The meeting, sponsored by WHO, UNAIDS, UNITAID and UNDP, focussed on identifying strategies and initiatives to overcoming the bottlenecks to increasing access to pharmaceutical technologies. Participants analysed ways to sustain treatment programmes and the scaling-up of coverage, ensure competition within the pharmaceutical sector and exceptions to intellectual property rights related to public health concerns.

The BRICS countries have a long history of making use of policy options, such as compulsory licensing to find a better balance in managing intellectual property rights for public health. At the same time, the BRICS countries expressed a strong desire to collaborate to create favourable environments for fostering accessibility and enhancing the affordability of health products in BRICS and other low- and middle-income countries.

Quotes

'There is a need for a renewed dialogue on access to medicines and intellectual property to ensure that no one is left behind. Success in one country represents success for many others. The BRICS are in a good position to lead the way.'

Luiz Loures, UNAIDS Deputy Executive Director

'The BRICS countries should work together with other developing countries to define concrete cooperation formulas to access commodities and regulations.'

Arthur Chioro, Minister of Health of Brazil

'People can be killed by biological weapons and can be killed by no access to medicines; the results are the same.'

Aaron Motsoaledi, Minister of Health of South Africa

'We have set a national target to produce 90% of vital medicines in the Russian Federation. We call on international pharmaceutical companies to participate in this process.'

Oleg Salagay, Deputy Head of the Department of International and Public Affairs of Russia

'We should work together to protect the full flexibility of TRIPS, and we call on international society to support the efforts of the countries.'

Sh. C. K. Mishra, Additional Secretary of International Cooperation (IC)/International Health (IH), Ministry of Health & Family Welfare of India

'We need to establish cooperation programmes on research and development and innovative technologies. We would hope for WHO and UNAIDS to play a bigger role in promoting South–South cooperation in this area.'

Zhang Yang, Deputy Director of the International Cooperation of NHFPC of China

24 May 2014

⇨ The above information is reprinted with kind permission from UNAIDS. Please visit www.unaids.org for further information.

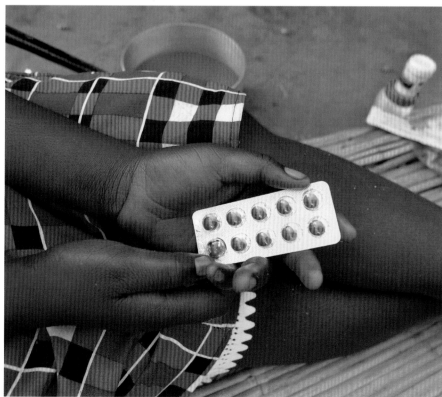

© UNAIDS 2014

Solving the toilet shortage needs a bottom-up approach

Why does one third of the world's population have inadequate sanitation?

By Dani Barrington

Hopefully I can shed a bit of light on this. You see, my work is shit – literally – which is why I call myself a water, sanitation and hygiene (WASH) engineer.

When people aren't completely scared off by my choice of discussion topics – such as faeces or the even more taboo menstrual hygiene management – they do often ask me why such a large proportion of the global population is still without adequate sanitation.

We, 'the experts', have already spent billions of dollars on this. So why haven't we succeeded in giving more people in developing countries access to toilets?

Well, we have tried: in the 1960s and 1970s, international aid was all about providing infrastructure. Here's a water treatment plant. Here's a toilet. Now go for your life.

But these often failed to consider the social, cultural, environmental and economic suitability and sustainability of different WASH interventions.

If you are used to relieving yourself in nature, why would you listen to these 'experts' telling you that it is 'healthier' to lock yourself in a small, foul-smelling box, even if it was given to you for free?

If you are an adolescent girl who has just started menstruating, is it useful for you to have a school toilet which provides no bins or washing facilities, and has to be shared with adolescent boys? Probably not.

What's 'appropriate'?

This is not to say that there aren't amazing things going on in WASH nowadays, thanks to programmes led by NGOs, governments, universities, industry and, probably most importantly, communities themselves.

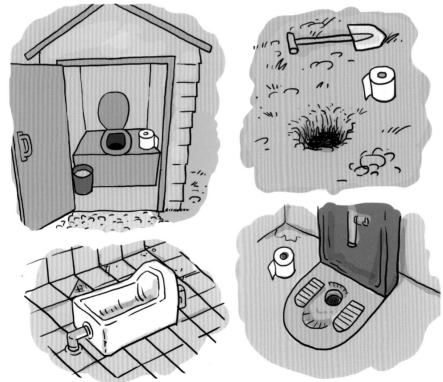

But it is not as simple as 'giving' people a toilet, or a tap, or tampons. A lot of the people to whom I speak assume that being a WASH engineer, I (and my colleagues) must have all the answers. We do not.

In most developing communities, the most appropriate technology is often quite modest and to be honest, in many cases the local users have much better skills than engineers at transforming WASH technologies to suit their own situations. Even the best university-taught skills aren't going to be particularly useful there.

Do I still have a job then?

Yes. WASH practitioners and researchers are now working on how they can ensure that WASH facilities, services and behaviours are sustainable and relevant in local contexts.

Giving someone access to a toilet or water source at some fixed point in time, which is how the UN currently measures the Millennium Development Goals for water and sanitation, does not imply that this will achieve 'sustainable access'.

If the users do not value the benefits, they will not use the facilities. If the users do not have the capacity or the resources to maintain and repair the systems, they will fall into disuse.

The development literature is riddled with examples. And even if a community does obtain 'sustainable access' to WASH facilities and services, do they really want them? Has access to these enhanced their health, self-worth, freedom and, ultimately, well-being?

Nobel Laureate Amartya Sen would certainly argue that development cannot be achieved without these. His seminal book *Development as Freedom* argues that without sufficient capabilities being attained and freedoms being met (including good health, stable finances, political freedom and access to opportunities), a person has not yet attained the well-being required to be considered 'developed'.

Participatory research methods have highlighted that outside 'experts' cannot walk into communities sprouting preconceived ideas of development: community members are the experts on their own lives.

The emphasis has shifted to building trust and rapport with these communities and giving them the support to develop workable solutions to address their immediate concerns.

This is where we can participate – by working alongside these communities and sharing our knowledge, be that in engineering, marketing, behaviour change or a myriad of other fields.

Communities bring their intimate knowledge of their own situations. It is through collaboration that we can help communities to improve their WASH facilities, services and behaviours, and develop their capacities, which, in turn, enhance their well-being.

It is no longer acceptable to simply assume that we know best – and, in my experience, the communities that I've worked with are not scared off when I start talking to them about toilet behaviours.

They tell me that their children are often sick with diarrhoea and they think that their WASH situation has something to do with it.

It is too important an issue to be labelled taboo.

Dr Dani Barrington works in the Department of Marketing at Monash University.

20 November 2013

⇨ The above information is reprinted with kind permission from Monash University. Please visit www.monash.edu for further information.

Fancy a toilet twin?

- Dorset-based charity Toilet Twinning works alongside communities all over the world to improve access to safe, hygienic sanitation facilities. For a £60 donation people can 'twin' their toilet with a latrine in:

  - Afghanistan
  - Bangladesh
  - Burundi
  - Cambodia
  - The Democratic Republic of Congo
  - India
  - Liberia
  - Sierra Leone
  - Uganda
  - Zambia

- Those who decide to donate receive a certificate of their toilet's 'twin', along with a photograph and GPS coordinates so they can look it up on Google Maps. Donations are used by Tearfund and Cord to 'enable local communities to learn about the difference a toilet will make to their lives', and improve the health of the community as a whole.

Visit www.toilettwinning.org for more information.

To fight malaria, we now have genetic weapons that can track and kill

An article from The Conversation.

By Sanjeev Krishna, Professor of Molecular Parasitology and Medicine at St George's, University of London

THE CONVERSATION

Every year malaria kills more than 600,000, which is a little less than the population of Bhutan. There are some simple solutions to control the disease, but keeping the numbers of mosquitoes with malarial parasites down remains a challenge.

The problem is that current control measures can wane in effectiveness as mosquitoes adapt. Discovering new ways to reduce mosquito numbers is therefore a high priority. An area where such advances are being made is genetics, and two recent studies are good examples of things to come.

Sex talk

Reducing the number of female mosquitoes, which are the transmitters of the malarial parasite, can drastically reduce the spread of the disease. In a study published in *Nature Communications*, researchers at Imperial College London are able to do that by using an enzyme that affects DNA.

Their laboratory results show that, within a few generations, whole colonies of mosquitoes can disappear when they use this enzyme. The enzyme selectively shreds the DNA of female mosquito, affecting those bits involved in reproduction (in particular, the X chromosome). Its offspring then are nearly

all male, leading to the collapse of the whole population.

Modifying the enzyme to damage the specific DNA took some time, and relied upon previous results that were initially obtained by curiosity-driven work. However, this new and successful application in the lab means field studies can begin soon.

Sleeping sickness in cattle, which is caused by tsetse flies, was eradicated from Zanzibar by the release of sterile male tsetse flies. But this was a costly and logistically demanding exercise that needed the saturation of a large area with nearly ten million sterile male flies produced by radiation treatment. The enzyme treatment might prove more cost effective, even though this is a different mosquito vector. It also gives more support to those in favour of genetic modification.

Genetic barcodes

Resistance to malarial drug patterns vary by geography. It would prove very useful if researchers are able to pinpoint the origin of a particular malarial strain, and researchers at the London School of Tropical Hygiene and Medicine have developed such a tool using genetic 'barcodes'.

To do this they analysed the genomes of more than 700 parasites found in Africa, Southeast Asia and Latin

America. Their report, also published in *Nature Communications*, found that most of the genome wasn't useful, but the bits of DNA in the mitochondria (the cell's powerhouse) and the apicoplast (a remnant of the plant cell found in the parasites) gave enough unique information to create a barcoding system.

The upshot of this quirk is that the barcoding system should last and get better as more genetic data is collected. This is because these bits of the DNA won't change much. They are passed down from mother to kids without recombining, unlike the rest of the DNA.

It is not enough to develop a new drug to replace a failing one, or discover another insecticide in the face of resistance in mosquitoes. Such imaginative technologies to reduce the enormous global footprint of malaria are needed. With genetic tools, we have taken the fight against malaria to the molecular level.

16 June 2014

⇨ The above information is reprinted with kind permission from The Conversation. Please visit www.theconversation.com for further information.

Millennium Development Goal (MDG) 6: combat HIV/AIDS, malaria and other diseases

Target 6A. *Have halted by 2015 and begun to reverse the spread of HIV/AIDS*

Target 6B. *Achieve, by 2010, universal access to treatment for HIV/AIDS for all those who need it.*

HIV/AIDS

At the end of 2012, 35.3million people were living with HIV. That same year, some 2.3 million people became newly infected, and 1.7 million died of AIDS, including 230 000 children. Close to ten million people in low- and middle-income countries were receiving antiretroviral therapy at the end of 2012. More than two-thirds of new HIV infections are in sub-Saharan Africa.

WHO is working with countries:

⇨ to prevent people becoming infected with HIV – helping to change behaviours to reduce HIV risks; increasing access to prevention commodities; supporting programmes for prevention of mother to child transmission of HIV; promoting safe blood supplies and prevention of HIV transmission in healthcare settings; assessing new prevention technologies;

⇨ to expand the availability of treatment;

⇨ to provide the best care for people living with HIV/AIDS and their families;

⇨ to expand access and uptake of HIV testing and counselling so that people can learn their HIV status;

⇨ to strengthen healthcare systems so that they can deliver quality and sustainable HIV/AIDS programmes and services; and

⇨ to improve HIV/AIDS information systems, including HIV surveillance, monitoring and evaluation and operational research.

Target 6C. *Have halted by 2015 and begun to reverse the incidence of malaria and other major diseases*

Malaria

Around the world, 3.3 billion people are at risk of contracting malaria. In 2012, an estimated 207 million cases occurred, and the disease killed approx. 627,000 people – most of them children under five in Africa. On average, malaria kills a child every minute.

WHO-recommended strategies to tackle malaria include:

⇨ prevention with long-lasting insecticidal nets and indoor residual spraying;

⇨ diagnostic testing and treatment with quality-assured anti-malarial medicines;

⇨ preventive therapies for infants, children and pregnant women;

⇨ tracking every malaria case in a surveillance system;

⇨ scaling up the fight against emerging drug and insecticide resistance.

In a 2007 resolution, the World Health Assembly called for a 75% reduction in the global malaria burden by 2015.

Tuberculosis

There were an estimated 8.6 million new cases of TB in 2012 (including 1.1 million cases among people with HIV) and an estimated 1.3 million deaths (including 320,000 people with HIV), making this disease one of the world's biggest infectious killers.

The world is on track to reach the MDG target of reversing TB incidence by 2015. However, incidence is falling very slowly. In addition, all regions, except Africa and Europe, are on track to achieve the Stop TB Partnership target of 50% decline in mortality by 2015.

WHO is working to combat the epidemic through the Stop TB Strategy. This six-point strategy seeks to:

⇨ pursue high-quality DOTS expansion and enhancement;

⇨ address TB/HIV, multidrug-resistant TB and the needs of poor and vulnerable populations;

⇨ contribute to health system strengthening based on primary health care;

⇨ engage all care providers;

⇨ empower people with TB, and communities through partnership; and

⇨ enable and promote research.

⇨ The above information is reprinted with kind permission from the World Health Organization. Please visit www.who.int for further information.

© WHO 2014

Ending newborn deaths: ensuring every baby survives

The first 24 hours of a child's life are the most dangerous, with more than one million babies dying each year on their first and only day of life, according to new research published by Save the Children.

The new report, *Ending Newborn Deaths*, shows one half of first day deaths around the world could be prevented if the mother and baby had access to free health care and a skilled midwife.

The children's aid agency says the deaths happen because of premature birth and complications during birth, such as prolonged labour, pre-eclampsia and infection, which can be avoided if quality health experts are present.

The research also found an additional 1.2 million babies are stillborn each year, their heartbeats stopping during labour because of childbirth complications, maternal infections and hypertension.

In a bid to save millions of newborn lives, Save the Children has called on world leaders to commit in 2014 to a blueprint for change – The Five Point Newborn Promise – which focusses on training and equipping enough skilled health workers to make sure no baby is born without proper help, and removing fees for all pregnancy and birth services.

The world has made amazing progress in reducing child mortality during the past decade – nearly halved from 12 million to 6.6 million – thanks to global political action on immunisation, treatment of pneumonia, diarrhoea, and malaria, family planning and nutrition.

But this progress could stall without urgent action to tackle scandalously high numbers of newborns dying. This report warns that newborn deaths now account for nearly half of all under-five deaths.

Carolyn Miles, President and CEO of Save the Children, said:

'The first day of a child's life is the most dangerous, and too many mothers give birth alone on the floor of their home or in the bush without any life-saving help. We hear horror stories of mothers walking for hours during labour to find trained help, all too often ending in tragedy.

'It's criminal that many of these deaths could be averted simply if there was someone on hand to make sure the birth took place safely and who knew what to do in a crisis.'

Each year, 40 million women give birth without trained help. In Ethiopia, only ten per cent of births have skilled help whereas in some areas of rural Afghanistan there is just one midwife for 10,000 people.

In countries such as the Democratic Republic of Congo (DRC) or the Central African Republic (CAR), some mothers have to pay for emergency maternal care, often costing as much as their monthly food bill. There have even been reports of mothers being kept under jail-like conditions for months until they have been able to pay for their emergency caesarean.

'More than one million babies die each year on their first and only day of life, according to new research published by Save the Children'

Carolyn Miles added: 'These new statistics reveal – for the first time ever – the true scale of the newborn crisis. The solutions are well-known but need greater political will to give babies a fighting chance of reaching their second day of life. Without targeted action now, progress made in cutting child mortality through vaccines and tackling malnutrition will stall.'

Save the Children is calling on world leaders, philanthropists and the private sector to meet and commit to the Five Point Newborn Promise in 2014:

⇨ Issue a defining and accountable declaration to end all preventable newborn mortality, saving two million newborn lives a year and stopping the 1.2 million stillbirths during labour

⇨ Ensure that by 2025 every birth is attended by trained and equipped health workers who can deliver essential newborn health interventions

⇨ Increase expenditure on health to at least the WHO minimum of US$60 per person

⇨ To pay for the training, equipping and support of health workers, and remove user fees for all maternal, newborn and child health services, including emergency obstetric care

⇨ The private sector, including pharmaceutical companies, should help address unmet needs by developing innovative solutions and increasing availability for the poorest to new and existing products for maternal, newborn and child health.

⇨ The above information is reprinted with kind permission from Save the Children. Please visit www.savethechildren.org for further information.

© Save the Children 2014

India shows the way for other polio-endemic nations

After India's unexpected feat of freeing itself from polio, the target to eradicate the debilitating disease from the world, set in 1988, seems possible.

By Kundan Pandey

When the WHO South East Asia region receives the certificate for being polio free on Thursday, it would be an accomplishment that until a few years ago was considered a pipe dream – mainly because of the large number of cases that continued to be reported from India.

As recently as 2009, India accounted for 741 out of the total 1,604 polio cases recorded across the world. While some experts believed that India would be the last country to be declared polio free, others said it was a task that could never be accomplished.

Eradication of the disease from India appeared to be the toughest part of the global campaign against the disease. There were several reasons for it: high density of population in India, poor sanitation, high birth rate, low rate of routine immunisation, widespread diarrhoea, difficult terrain, high rate of migration and also resistance to vaccination among some groups.

In spite of these hurdles, India did manage to overcome the challenge and was declared polio free this year after no case was reported for three consecutive years. Celebrating the achievement on 11 February, director-general of the World Health Organization (WHO), Margaret Chan, said that many critics believed that this day would never come, that the polio virus was too firmly entrenched in India, and that India would never be polio free.

The global threat

But the risk is not gone as yet. The polio-free status of every country is under threat as long as poliovirus is prevalent in any part of the world. According to Bill & Melinda Gates Foundation, more than 20 countries have experienced outbreaks of polio, imported from endemic countries – some of them multiple times – since 2008.

After South East Asia gets the certificate on Thursday, only two regions, East Mediterranean and Africa, will be left out of list of polio-free certified regions. The remaining three WHO regions are: Americas (got certificate in 1994), European region (2002) and Western Pacific region (2000).

After India's unexpected feat, the target to eradicate polio from the world, set in 1988, seems possible. It is believed that the other two regions are not as difficult as India was. Moreover, India is assisting countries, including Pakistan, Afghanistan (East Mediterranean region) and Nigeria (Africa). This is expected to make the task less difficult.

Lessons to learn from India's achievement

The story of India's victory against polio involves fight against challenges like surveillance, confusion over separate pockets, infrastructure issues, logistical limitations and dealing with marginalised groups. India's collaboration with international agencies like WHO, Rotary international and Unicef made it possible to achieve the feat.

When India faced the problem of identifying children in need of vaccination, National Polio Surveillance Project was established in 1997. The government included community leaders to deal with local challenges. In an interview with Down To Earth, WHO regional director for South-East Asia, Poonam Khetrapal Singh, said, 'Success in eradicating polio has come after intensive community involvement. Working with local, traditional and religious leaders in advocating the benefits of the vaccination helps fight false perceptions and build confidence in immunisation.' It is well-known that Bollywood star Amitabh Bachhan was also roped in for the immunisation campaign because of his influence on people.

To reach the hidden pockets, local people and health workers were engaged. This helped to trace even those children who had never been targeted by any other health programme. Tracking such groups not only helped in eradicating polio but may also help in other health campaigns in future.

For other countries which are still suffering from polio, Khetrapal said that there are many lessons to learn from the experience of India. It includes ensuring accountability at every level of administration for delivering service to the community. She also suggested that it is important to focus on finding local solutions to solve local challenges. It may need some innovations, technologies and mapping to ensure vaccination of migrant communities.

27 March 2014

⇨ The above information is reprinted with kind permission from Down To Earth. Please visit www.downtoearth.org.in for further information.

Key facts

⇨ Based on global averages, a girl who was born in 2012 can expect to live to around 73 years and a boy to the age of 68. (page 1)

⇨ The top six countries where life expectancy increased the most were Liberia which saw a 20-year increase (from 42 years in 1990 to 62 years in 2012) followed by Ethiopia (from 45 to 64 years), Maldives (58 to 77 years), Cambodia (54 to 72 years), Timor-Leste (50 to 66 years) and Rwanda (48 to 65 years). (page 1)

⇨ Life expectancy for both men and women is still less than 55 years in nine sub-Saharan African countries – Angola, Central African Republic, Chad, Côte d'Ivoire, Democratic Republic of the Congo, Lesotho, Mozambique, Nigeria and Sierra Leone. (page 1)

⇨ Around 44 million (6.7%) of the world's children aged less than five years were overweight or obese in 2012. Ten million of these children were in the WHO African Region where levels of child obesity have increased rapidly. (page 2)

⇨ Globally, the number of new HIV infections continues to fall. There were 2.3 million new HIV infections [1.9 million–2.7 million] in 2012. This is the lowest number of annual new infections since the mid-to-late 1990s, when approximately 3.5 million [3.3 million–4.1 million] people were acquiring HIV every year. (page 4)

⇨ Out of the global total of 35.3 million [32.2 million–38.8 million] people living with HIV, an estimated 3.6 million [3.2 million–3.9 million] are people aged 50 years or older. (page 4)

⇨ Britain is now the only nation in Western Europe with rising levels of tuberculosis, with more than 9,000 cases diagnosed annually. In London, where 40% of UK cases are reportedly diagnosed, the number of cases has risen by almost 50% since 1999, up from 2,309 in 1999 to 3,450 in 2009. (page 5)

⇨ One in 200 [polio] infections leads to irreversible paralysis, usually in the legs. This is caused by the virus entering the bloodstream and invading the central nervous system. As it multiplies, the virus destroys the nerve cells that activate muscles. The affected muscles are no longer functional and the limb becomes floppy and lifeless – a condition known as acute flaccid paralysis (AFP). (page 9)

⇨ Ebola was first identified in Africa in the mid-1970s. An outbreak that began in March 2014 was the most serious so far. By 13 August 2014 it had killed more than 1,000 people across Guinea, Liberia, Sierra Leone and Nigeria. (page 10)

⇨ According to studies from eight countries, an average dengue episode represents 14.8 lost days for ambulatory patients at an average cost of US$514 and 18.9 days for non-fatal hospitalised patients at an average cost of US$1491. (page 12)

⇨ NCDs kill 36 million people a year – more than all other causes combined. They are the most frequent cause of death in most countries and account for nearly two thirds of all deaths globally. If current trends continue, NCD deaths will increase by 15 per cent over the next decade, reaching 44 million a year. (page 15)

⇨ According to the World Health Organization (WHO), cholera affects three to five million people worldwide and causes between 100,000 and 130,000 deaths per year. (page 18)

⇨ Gout admissions have increased by a fifth since 2009–10 in England, with almost 5,800 admissions in the 12 months to April 2014. The latest gout admissions figure is a four per cent rise on the previous 12-month period (5,560) and a 22 per cent rise since 2009–10 (4,760). (page 20)

⇨ Over the last five years there was a 71 per cent increase in hospital admissions where malnutrition was a primary or secondary diagnosis, from 3,900 admissions in 2009–10 to 6,690 admissions in 2013–14. (page 20)

⇨ On any given day in Australia, about 40 per cent of hospital in-patients will receive antibiotics, with between 20 and 50 per cent of those deemed unnecessary or sub-optimal in current best practice terms, depending on the individual hospital. (page 26)

⇨ NHS figures show that the prescription of antibiotic drugs has increased by 30% since the year 2000, and an estimated 5,000 people die each year because of drug-resistant strains of bacteria. (page 27)

⇨ There are still 2.5 billion people, or over one third of the world's population, without access to adequate sanitation. (page 31)

⇨ Around 700,000 children die every year from diarrhoea caused by unsafe water and poor sanitation. That's almost 2,000 children a day. (page 31)

⇨ As recently as 2009, India accounted for 741 out of the total 1,604 polio cases recorded across the world but in 2014 it was declared polio free after three consecutive years with no cases reported. (page 39)

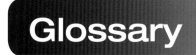

AIDS

Acquired Immune Deficiency Syndrome. AIDS is a potentially fatal illness. It develops at the most advanced stage of HIV.

Antimicrobial resistance

A broad term used to refer to 'drug resistance' where a microbe or virus becomes resistant or immune to the drugs used to treat it. Doctors are increasingly concerned that over-prescription of antibiotics has led to some people developing a resistance which means the drugs are less effective.

Cholera

An infectious disease that affects the small intestine. Cholera is usually contracted from infected water supplies and causes extreme sickness and diarrhoea.

Communicable diseases

Diseases that you can catch from another person or being. Also known as 'infectious' diseases.

Ebola

An infectious and usually fatal disease that is characterised by severe fever and internal bleeding. It is spread through contact with infected bodily fluids.

Malaria

A life-threatening disease caused by a parasite that is transmitted by *Anopheles* mosquito. With correct medication and precautions, Malaria is preventable and treatable. Only the female *Anopheles* mosquito can transmit the disease to a human.

Millennium Development Goals

The world's targets for addressing poverty, education, disease, equality and environmental sustainability.

Non-communicable diseases (NCDs)

These diseases cannot be transmitted from person to person, e.g. heart disease.

Obesity

When someone is obese, they have a BMI of 30 or over. This puts them at risk for a number of serious health problems, such as an increased risk of heart disease and type 2 diabetes. Worldwide obesity has more than doubled since 1980 and this is most likely due to our more sedentary lifestyle, combined with a lack of physical exercise.

Sanitation

Usually refers to access to clean drinking water and adequate sewage facilities.

Tuberculosis

An infectious disease, usually known as TB. TB involves a bacterial infection that spreads through the lymph nodes to different organs in the body; most often the lungs. TB often shows no signs or symptoms until the immune system weakens and the bacteria becomes active.

Vector-borne diseases

Diseases that are transmitted among humans or animals, usually by insects. Malaria is an example of a vector-borne disease because it is transmitted by mosquitoes.

World Health Organization (WHO)

WHO is an agency of the United Nations (UN) that is dedicated to global public health issues.

Zoonotic diseases

Diseases spread between animals and humans, e.g. rabies.

Assignments

campaign could include posters, TV adverts, radio adverts, social media marketing or website banners.

Brainstorming

⇨ In small groups, discuss what you know about global health. Consider the following points:

- What global health issues can you think of?
- What is the difference between communicable and non-communicable diseases?
- What are vector-borne diseases?
- What do the Millennium Development Goals say about global health?

Research

⇨ Create a questionnaire to find out how much your class knows about antibiotics and what they can treat. Write a report that analyses your findings and include at least three graphs or infographics to illustrate your information.

⇨ Read the article on page 28 and conduct some further research into illnesses caused by air pollution. Write some notes and feedback to your class.

⇨ Choose a country from the map on page 16 and research the cultural factors that might relate to their leading cause of death.

⇨ Choose one of the diseases discussed in this book and research its history and the development of related treatments. Write a summary of your findings, or design a timeline.

⇨ Worldwide, the top cause of premature death is heart disease. Research contributing factors and then, as a class, discuss how people can reduce their risk of developing heart disease.

Design

⇨ Look at the *Life expectancy at birth* table on page 1 and design a graph, map or infographic to illustrate the statistics.

⇨ Design a poster that promotes the steps you can take to protect yourself from malaria when travelling abroad.

⇨ Choose one of the articles in this book and create an illustration to highlight the key themes/message of your chosen article.

⇨ Imagine you work for a charity that promotes water, sanitation and hygiene in developing countries. Design a campaign to raise awareness of how these issues affect women and girls. Your

Oral

⇨ As a class, discuss what you think could be done to prevent the obesity crisis in Africa. How could you inform people about the health risks of eating westernised food such as McDonald's?

⇨ Research polio and create a five-minute presentation explaining its causes, treatment and the history of the disease.

⇨ Create a presentation that will persuade people in your local community to 'twin' their toilet (see page 35).

⇨ In small groups, discuss what you have been taught about AIDS and HIV at school. Create a detailed plan for a lesson that will teach pupils of your age-group from developing countries in Africa about these illnesses. Think carefully about what should be included and consider how you will make the lesson interesting, memorable and relevant to their circumstances.

Reading/writing

⇨ Write an article exploring the recent outbreaks of Ebola virus and what is being done to treat and prevent its spread. Write no more than 1,000 words.

⇨ Write a blog post that explores zoonotic diseases – you could focus on the topic as a whole or choose one particular disease.

⇨ Write a one-paragraph definition of non-communicable diseases.

⇨ Read the article *New analysis shows current picture of diseases which were widespread in the Victorian era* on page 20 and write a summary for your school newspaper.

⇨ Write a diary entry from the perspective of a girl or woman living in a village where there is no access to proper sanitation or toilets.

⇨ Watch the 2011 film *Contagion* and write a review exploring how the director deals with the theme of widespread disease.

Acknowledgements

The publisher is grateful for permission to reproduce the material in this book. While every care has been taken to trace and acknowledge copyright, the publisher tenders its apology for any accidental infringement or where copyright has proved untraceable. The publisher would be pleased to come to a suitable arrangement in any such case with the rightful owner.

Images

Cover and pages iii, 15 and 33: iStock. Pages 13 and 23: Morguefile. Page 14 © Rick Scavetta, U.S. Army Africa, reproduced under creative commons license (https://creativecommons.org/licenses/by/2.0/). Page 26 © Jackie Staines. Page 31: Department of Foreign Affairs and Trade, Australian Government (Flickr).

Icons used on pages 2, 32, 35 are courtesy of Freepik. Icon on page 41 © SimpleIcon.

Illustrations

Don Hatcher: pages 20 & 36. Simon Kneebone: pages 6 & 28. Angelo Madrid: pages 18 & 34.

Additional acknowledgements

Editorial on behalf of Independence Educational Publishers by Cara Acred.

With thanks to the Independence team: Mary Chapman, Sandra Dennis, Christina Hughes, Jackie Staines and Jan Sunderland.

Cara Acred

Cambridge

January 2015